Drug Development Life Cycle

Edited by Juber Akhtar, Badruddeen, Mohammad Ahmad and Mohammad Irfan Khan

Published in London, United Kingdom

Drug Development Life Cycle
http://dx.doi.org/10.5772/intechopen.96842
Edited by Juber Akhtar, Badruddeen, Mohammad Ahmad and Mohammad Irfan Khan

Contributors
Neelima Dhingra, Anupam Nath Jha, Subhomoi Borkotoky, Amit Joshi, Vikas Kaushik, Juber Akhtar, Nazneen Sultana, Badruddeen, Mohammad Irfan Khan, Usama Ahmad, Muhammad Arif, Mohammad Ahmad, Tanmay Upadhyay, Zahra Rezaei, Behnaz Eslami, Rajendra Jangde, Prakriti Diwan, Sulekha Khunte, Harish Bhardwaj, Preeti K. Suresh

First published in London, United Kingdom, 2022 by IntechOpen
IntechOpen is the global imprint of INTECHOPEN LIMITED, registered in England and Wales, registration number: 11086078, 5 Princes Gate Court, London, SW7 2QJ, United Kingdom

British Library Cataloguing-in-Publication Data
A catalogue record for this book is available from the British Library

Additional hard and PDF copies can be obtained from orders@intechopen.com

Drug Development Life Cycle
Edited by Juber Akhtar, Badruddeen, Mohammad Ahmad and Mohammad Irfan Khan
p. cm.
Print ISBN 978-1-80356-047-2
Online ISBN 978-1-80356-048-9
eBook (PDF) ISBN 978-1-80356-049-6

Meet the editors

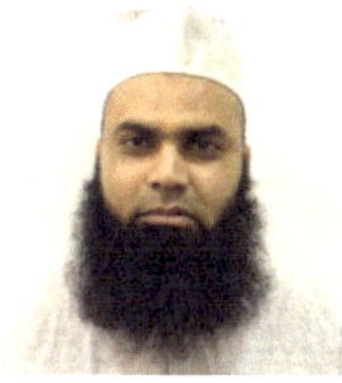

Dr. Juber Akhtar has more than 15 years of research and teaching experience. He obtained his BPharm and MPharm from Jamia Hamdard, New Delhi, India, and Manipal University, Karnataka, India. He obtained his Ph.D. from Integral University, Lucknow, India. Dr. Akhtar was nominated as the head of the Faculty of Pharmacy, at Integral University. He also served as chairman cum biological scientist for the Institutional Animal Ethics Committee (IAEC). He is a member of the Causality Assessment Committee (CAC) and the Animal House facility, at Integral University. He has experience teaching abroad and was previously a professor at Buraydah College of Pharmacy and Dentistry, Kingdom of Saudi Arabia (KSA). Dr. Akhtar has more than ninety publications in reputed journals to his credit. He is an academic book editor and an editorial board member for many esteemed journals. He has supervised a dozen Ph.D. and MPharm students in research projects. Dr. Akhtar's areas of research interest include the development of nanoparticulate drug delivery systems.

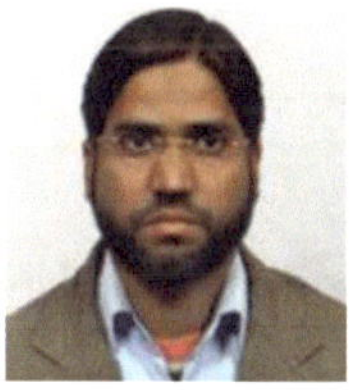

Dr. Badruddeen obtained both a BPharm and MPharm from Hamdard University, Delhi, India. He obtained a Ph.D. in Pharmacology from Integral University, Lucknow, India, in 2014. He has expertise in cardiovascular, neurodegenerative, and endocrine diseases. He has experience in conducting research on the safety, toxicity, and clinical efficacy of herbal and allopathic drugs. He has many original articles in reputed journals to his credit. Dr. Badruddeen is an academic book editor and an editorial board member for many esteemed journals. He has supervised a dozen research scholars and is a member of the Indian Science Congress Association, member secretary of the Institutional Animal Ethics Committee (IAEC), coordinator of the Adverse Drug Monitoring Center (AMC), chairman of the Causality Assessment Committee (CAC), and a member of the Animal House facility, Integral University.

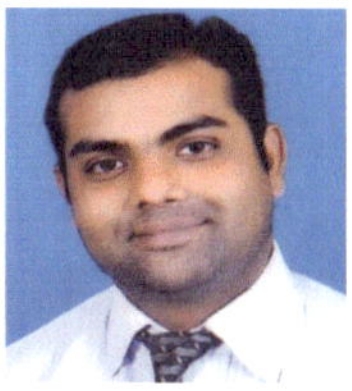

Dr. Mohammad Irfan Khan obtained an MPharm from Hamdard University, Delhi, India. He obtained his Ph.D. in Phytochemistry from Singhania University, Jhunjhunu, India. He has expertise in Ayurvedic medicine and nutraceuticals and has worked with some of the world's major pharmaceutical companies. He has more than 12 years of experience in research and formulation development of Ayurvedic, herbal, and nutraceutical products and successfully developed more than 100 formulations. He has more than forty original papers in international journals to his credit. Dr. Khan has supervised many research scholars at the post-graduate and Ph.D. levels.

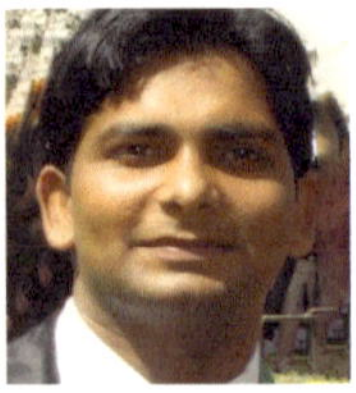

Dr. Mohammad Ahmad holds a specialization in Pharmacology from Jamia Hamdard, New Delhi, India. He received his Ph.D. from Integral University, Lucknow, India. Presently, he is an Assistant Professor of Pharmacology, at the Faculty of Pharmacy, at Integral University. He has been teaching PharmD, BPharm, and MPharm students and conducting research in the field of diabetes and cancer. From 2011 to 2014, he worked as a research assistant on a project sponsored by the Council for Science and Technology, Uttar Pradesh, India. He has published more than twenty original articles in reputed journals. He is a member of the British Society of Nanomedicine, Indian Science Congress Association, and International NanoScience Community, Budapest, Hungry. He is also a social nominee of the Committee for the Purpose of Control and Supervision of Experiments on Animals (CPCSEA). Dr. Ahmad is actively involved in research and his areas of interest include pharmacology and drug and pharmaceutical regulatory affairs. He is also engaged in research pertaining to diabetes mellitus, oral delivery of anticancer agents, and chemoprevention using natural bioactive compounds.

Contents

Preface

The development of a new drug product or biologic is an extended, multifarious, and costly progression that usually takes on an average 10 to 12 years. Occasionally, extra time may be required from product development to commercialization. This book presents a comprehensive overview of drug design, highlighting the steps involved from the discovery phase to product approval.

The book is divided into four sections. Section 1 discusses drug development, highlighting analytical processes, some adverse drug reactions associated with drugs in a few conditions, and repurposing of medicaments in various ailments. Section 2 discusses the topical application of drugs. It includes some pharmaceutical nanoformulations and cosmeceuticals useful in various diseases including topical diseases. Section 3 focuses on ocular drug delivery systems and the barriers encountered during the delivery of drugs in the eyes. Section 4 explores *in silico* drug development involving computer-aided drug design, machine learning, and artificial intelligence. It also examines the computational and statistical methods used to investigate and analyze chemicals in pharmaceutical medicine.

This book is written by experts in the field and is a useful resource for students, researchers, and academicians. I am thankful to all the authors for their excellent contributions.

Dr. Juber Akhtar
Associate Professor,
Faculty of Pharmacy,
Integral University,
Lucknow, India

Badruddeen, Mohammad Irfan Khan and Mohammad Ahmad
Integral University,
Lucknow, India

Section 1

Investigation of Medicine Progress

Chapter 1

Introductory Chapter: Drug Development Life Cycle

Juber Akhtar and Badruddeen

1. Introduction

Drug development comprises all the activities involved in transforming a compound from drug candidate (the end product of the discovery phase) to a product approved for marketing, that is, the dosage form which will be available in the market for sale after the approval of the appropriate regulatory authorities (**Figure 1**).

2. Topical formulations

The drug development of topical formulations involving nanoemulgel delivery system in which fusion of two different delivery systems and the physical state of drug containing nanoemulsion is elaborated. A nanoemulsion which is a thermodynamically stable system might be transformed into the nanogel. A formulator thus can make the incorporation of lipophilic drugs in the system and further might be used in treatment. The poor oral bioavailability, and unpredictable pharmacokinetic and absorption variation of various drugs can be overcome by this technique. Simultaneously, its non-greasy nature and easily spreading ability support the patient compliance. The treatment of acne, pimple, psoriasis, fungal infection, and inflammation caused by osteoarthritis and rheumatoid arthritis is possible.

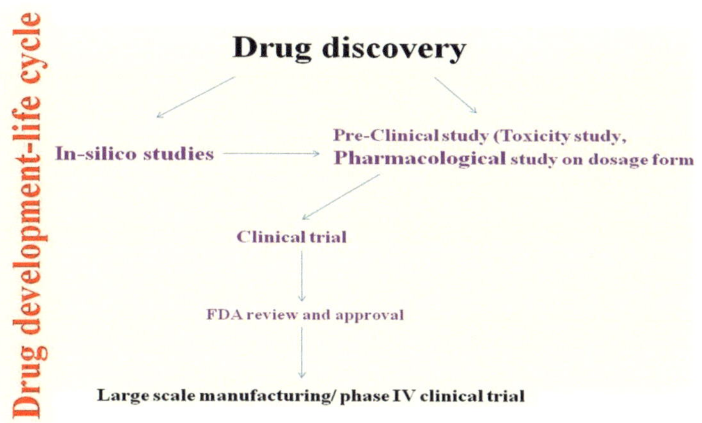

Figure 1.
A brief summary on drug development.

3. The ophthalmic preparations

The ophthalmic preparations and various barriers affecting drug penetration and distribution inside the eye were also explained. As per World Health Organization, the prevalence of distance or near vision impairment is increasing. Both the anterior and posterior areas of the eyes are affected by various degenerative infections. These may be age-related macular degeneration and diabetic retinopathy at the posterior segment, which can cause severe vision loss. The ocular drug delivery is one of the challenges for delivery of medicaments since it has number of anatomical and physiological barriers. Keeping in mind one full chapter has been compiled in the book in which various barriers that can protect the external and internal structures of the eye from the passage of drugs are elaborated. However, it is very difficult to attain effective pharmacotherapy because of these barriers. Many conventional dosage forms (eye drops and ointments) cannot achieve therapeutic concentrations in the posterior region of eye since only an extremely small amount of drug (1/100,000) can reach the retina and choroid. Although investigations into novel dosage forms that can be applied topically are underway, the topical dosage form might be formed and may target posterior segment diseases [1, 2].

4. The machine learning and artificial intelligence and computer-aided drug design (CADD)

The machine learning and artificial intelligence (AI) and computer-aided drug design (CADD) are also the new challenges for formulation developer. One can identify and practically implement the number of computational and statistical methods for analyzing biomedical entities, so that target identification will be easy, cost-effective, and validated ones. To complete the drug development processes, CADD can be used to attain biochemical safety and effectiveness, and to stay away from toxicity. The *in silico* techniques that are accepted in academics, firms, and administration [3, 4] may lead to momentous improvement in drug blueprint and innovations. Since a huge raw data (primary data) were obtained during and after biological, chemical, and pharmaceutical medicine development, there is need of machine learning algorithms that can be optimized and same to be applied in the countryside of CADD. In this way, significant improvement in the competence of drug design and discovery processes is possible. If a formulator apply computational methods and tools during drug design and discovery and development, one can think over an accurate and reliable pre-processed data [5, 6]. Further artificial intelligence (AI) approaches might be useful for pre-processing of huge data [7] and its modeling [8, 9] and overall design of the dosage forms.

Author details

Juber Akhtar* and Badruddeen
Faculty of Pharmacy, Integral University, Lucknow, India

*Address all correspondence to: jakhtar@iul.ac.in

References

[1] Lee J, Rhee YS. Ophthalmic dosage forms for drug delivery to posterior segment. Journal of Pharmaceutical Investigation. 2022;**52**:161-173

[2] Loftsson T. Topical drug delivery to the retina: Obstacles and routes to success. Expert Opinion on Drug Delivery. 2022;**19**(1):9-21

[3] Schaduangrat N, Lampa S, Simeon S, Gleeson MP, Spjuth O, Nantasenamat C. Towards reproducible computational drug discovery. Journal of Cheminformatics. 2020;**12**:9. DOI: 10.1186/s13321-020-0408-x

[4] Yang X, Wang YF, Byrne R, Schneider G, Yang SY. Concepts of artificial intelligence for computer-assisted drug discovery. Chemical Reviews. 2019;**119**:10520-10594. DOI: 10.1021/acs.chemrev.8b00728

[5] Katsila T, Spyroulias GA, Patrinos GP, Matsoukas MT. Computational approaches in target identification and drug discovery. Computational and Structural Biotechnology Journal. 2016;**14**:177-184. DOI: 10.1016/j.csbj.2016.04.004

[6] Macalino SJY, Gosu V, Hong SH, Choi S. Role of computer-aided drug design in modern drug discovery. Archives of Pharmacal Research. 2015;**38**:1686-1701. DOI: 10.1007/s12272-015-0640-5

[7] Hu YH, Lin WC, Tsai CF, Ke SW, Chen CW. An efficient data preprocessing approach for large scale medical data mining. Technology and Health Care. 2015;**23**:153-160. DOI: 10.3233/THC-140887

[8] Car J, Sheikh A, Wicks P, Williams MS. Beyond the hype of big data and artificial intelligence: Building foundations for knowledge and wisdom. BMC Medicine. 2019;**17**:143. DOI: 10.1186/s12916-019-1382-x

[9] Saez C, Garcia-Gomez JM. Kinematics of big biomedical data to characterize temporal variability and seasonality of data repositories: Functional data analysis of data temporal evolution over non-parametric statistical manifolds. International Journal of Medical Informatics. 2018;**119**:109-124. DOI: 10.1016/j.ijmedinf.2018.09.015

Chapter 2

A Method for Plotting Disease Drug Analysis and Its Complications by Combining Sources of Scientific Documents Using Deep Learning Method with Drug Repurposing: Case Study Metformin

Zahra Rezaei and Behnaz Eslami

Abstract

Drugs for medical purposes aim at saving one's life and improving their life quality. Side effects or adverse drug reactions (ADRs) on patients are studied as an important issue in pharmacology. In order to prevent the adverse drug effects, clinical trials are conducted on the drug production process, but the process of these trials is very costly and time consuming. So, various text mining methods are used to identify ADRs on scientific documents and articles. Using existing articles in the reference websites such as PubMed to predict an effective drug in the disease is a vital way to declare the drug effective. However, the effective integration of biomedical literature and biological drug network information is one of the major challenges in diagnosing a new drug. In this study, we use medical text documents to train the BioBERT model so that we can use it to discover potential drugs for treating diseases. Then, we are able to create a graphical network of drugs and their side effects with this method as well as it provides us with an opportunity to identify effective drugs that have been used in many diseases so far while having the ability to be used effectively on other diseases.

Keywords: adverse drug reactions, drug repurposing, deep learning, natural language processing, social network

1. Introduction

What makes reusing old drugs worthwhile is the cost of developing a new drug, according to research [1]. The cost of developing a new drug reaches billions of dollars, which includes analysis, testing, validation costs, and so on. More importantly, duration of developing new drugs may take long nearly 9 to 12 years to launch a new drug.

This practice, therefore, is deemed to be of importance in the pharmaceutical industry because it accelerates the development of drugs and reduces the cost of drug production, especially for pandemic diseases such as COVID-19, and the need to use this scientific process in the field of artificial intelligence is essential.

Due to the rapid growth of scientific articles in medical research, the analysis of medical textual documents using text mining methods has become very popular. The emergence of powerful deep learning methods and their maturity in text mining has created various development ways for different types of text analysis. The only drawback of deep learning models is their training using a large number of input data, which has made an unsurmountable challenge in medical topics. Fortunately, various medical sites such as PubMed allow the use of textual data and have seriously contributed to the development of deep learning models.

Improvements in healthcare and nutrition have generated remarkable increases in life expectancy worldwide. Although our understanding of the molecular basis of these morbidities has quickly advanced, effective novel treatments are still lacking. Today, the topic of reusing drugs based on text mining methods and based on valid scientific articles is important and vital, because based on the characteristics of pharmacokinetics and pharmacodynamics, the process of data generation has already been approved and validated by scientific communities and the study of side effects, and their impact on other diseases will significantly save the time and cost of the data generation process. Creating new drug profiles based on previously valid drugs is a way of bypassing the drug production cycle.

Metformin is one such drug currently being investigated for novel applications.

What is clear from the clinical evidence is that metformin is prescribed in the treatment of diabetes. The aim of this research is to investigate the effects of metformin on various diseases that are reflected in PubMed documents. What will be studied in this report are the results of the use of metformin in the prevention of various diseases.

This chapter aims to provide the reported results, available in medical literatures for potential of metformin to prevent or treat different kinds of disorders.

Furthermore, some of the previous researches in the field of drug reuse have been reviewed in the second chapter. In the third chapter, the proposed research model is discussed and in the fourth chapter, the explanation of the model architecture is discussed. The implementation results and final outputs of the proposed method are explained in the last section.

2. Related works

Drug reuse is used to treat diseases other than an approved disease (such as drug use in new drugs, development of indications, or change of indications), including the development of new medical applications for previously approved drugs, as well as the evolutionary cycle. A drug is defined for the use and development of drugs that are in the drug archive. This strategy is not very new, but it has gained significant momentum in the last decade as approved scientific sources on drug reuse have identified side effects.

About one-third of the approvals in recent years correspond to drug repurposing, and repurposed drugs currently generate around 25% of the annual revenue for the pharmaceutical industry [2].

Drug reuse involves identifying new uses for existing drugs. Prominent examples of the use of these methods include sildenafil and thalidomide as a result of serendipity [3].

Graphs of drugs, genes, and diseases are created and clustering methods are developed to predict new edges between drugs and diseases [4].

Disease genes and drug genes are modeled. Relationships from Medical Scientific Documents and Induction of Indirect Relationships Between Drugs and Diseases Proposed a ranking method based on the similarity of the drug target to rank these relationships [5].

When predicting a new drug-target interactions (DTI), drug-drug interaction (DDI) [6], there are three levels of prediction using machine learning techniques. First, it preprocesses input data such as drug side effects, drug chemical structure, and disease genes and provides training data through feature extraction. The appropriate machine learning algorithm is then used for training. Third, we apply a predictive model to get the results of drug repositioning in the test dataset. The data is transformed into a consistent, normalized format, such as computer-readable vectors and matrices, before being entered into the machine learning model to train the representation. Representation learning [7] (or feature learning) is a set of techniques for transforming raw data into something that can be effectively used through machine learning. Representation learning is mainly divided into a supervised learning approach and an unsupervised learning approach and extracts the properties of the input data of the downstream.

3. Material and methods

We look for relevant publication in PubMed through using metformin as key word. The data of this research are documents and scientific articles written in English between 1994 and 2020. In this direction, we applied named entity recognition (NER) BioBERT method.

The used NER method includes three main phases (**Figure 1**); it is started with textual documents from PubMed which are entered as input data, followed by preprocessing phase to improve data, and eventually, in the third phase, grouping data into train and test categories is done, and NER via deep learning algorithm – BioBERT method – runs to extract patterns.

3.1 Data sources

We looked at 18000 publications in PubMed using metformin as a keyword. The abstracts of 16,000 out of them were analyzed by NER BioBERT. This search covered studies which have been done between 1994 and 2020.

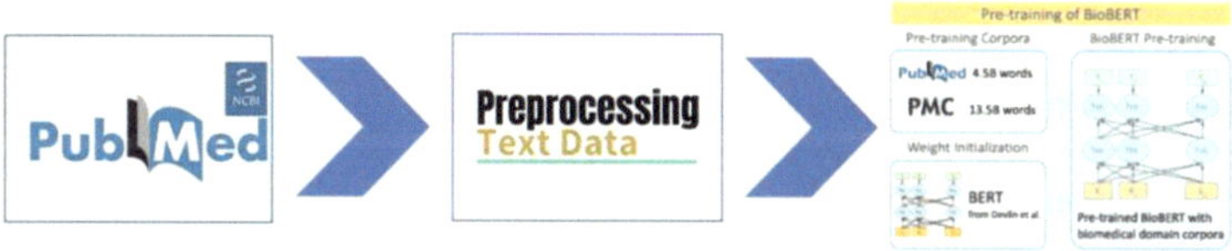

Figure 1.
The workflow of the proposed model-based strategy.

3.2 Preprocessing

The preprocessing of comments in both datasets was performed as follows:

1. Data shuffling
2. Converting all uppercase words into lowercase
3. Elimination of special characters such as @,!, /, *, $.
4. Remove stop words such as at, of, the.
5. Convert acronym or abbreviation to complete
6. Lemmatization

3.3 Deep classification

Bidirectional Encoder Representations from Transformers for Biomedical Text Mining can be considered a particular language pretrained model on a large-scale biomedical corpus. According to the mentioned architecture, the knowledge from a large number of biomedical documents by BioBERT [8] is transferred to biomedical text mining models with the least amount of modification in the architecture. Whereas competitive performances with previous novel models appeared by BERT and BIOBERT essentially have better performance on the following three biomedical text mining functions: biomedical named entity recognition and biomedical clustering based on the effect of Metformin.

Different diseases and the trend of metformin impact in publication during several years, based on drug effect on various diseases.

BioBERT effectively moved the data from a part of biomedical textual documents to biomedical text mining models by some alterations in a particular structure. Whereas BERT had outlined excellent function with previous models, BioBERT discernibly overwhelmed them on entity recognition and clustering concerning metformin effect on individuals' wellbeing.

We investigated publications based on the association between metformin and type 1 and 2 diabetes. And separately, we explored them in accordance with the effect of metformin on other disease.

PubTator [9] and BEST [10] are two of the potential sources that automatically can extract compounds and proteins from PubMed or PubMed Central (PMC). However, these two sources are not able to extract the combined and interactive relationships between the drug and the disease. To address these issues, we began building a pipeline using NER to identify studies containing DTI and extract related data. We, then, trained the BioBERT model on known studies containing DTIs and used this model to predict new drug studies.

Indeed, given an input sentence X = {x1, x2, ..., xN} where x_i is the i-th word/token and N speaks to the length of the sentence. The objective of NER is to categorize each word/token in X and allot it to corresponding name y ϵ Y, where Y may be a predefined list of all conceivable name sorts (e.g. CHEMICAL as Drugs, Infection).

Additionally, this structure was used after preprocessing to identify the relationship between the drug and the disease. In future research, we are going to create this graph of relationships and use the number of drug references to a chemical structure as a weight to discover drug relationships.

4. Result

There have been a few detailed examinations into the relationship between metformin and the results of cures in different diseases. Moreover, these preclinical reports and dependable biological pathways have been known which clarify the atomic component of metformin and addressed in our research work. Nevertheless, the vital reply to this issue is the level of metformin adequacy against nondiabetic disarranges.

Metformin is the generic name of the drug which is produced and supplied under different brand names such as Metformex, Glucophage, and so on. As shown in **Figure 2**, the drugs extracted from the authoritative scientific articles are in the drug groups related to diabetes and some other drug groups.There are several classes of drugs used to control diabetes, and members belonging to each group have similar

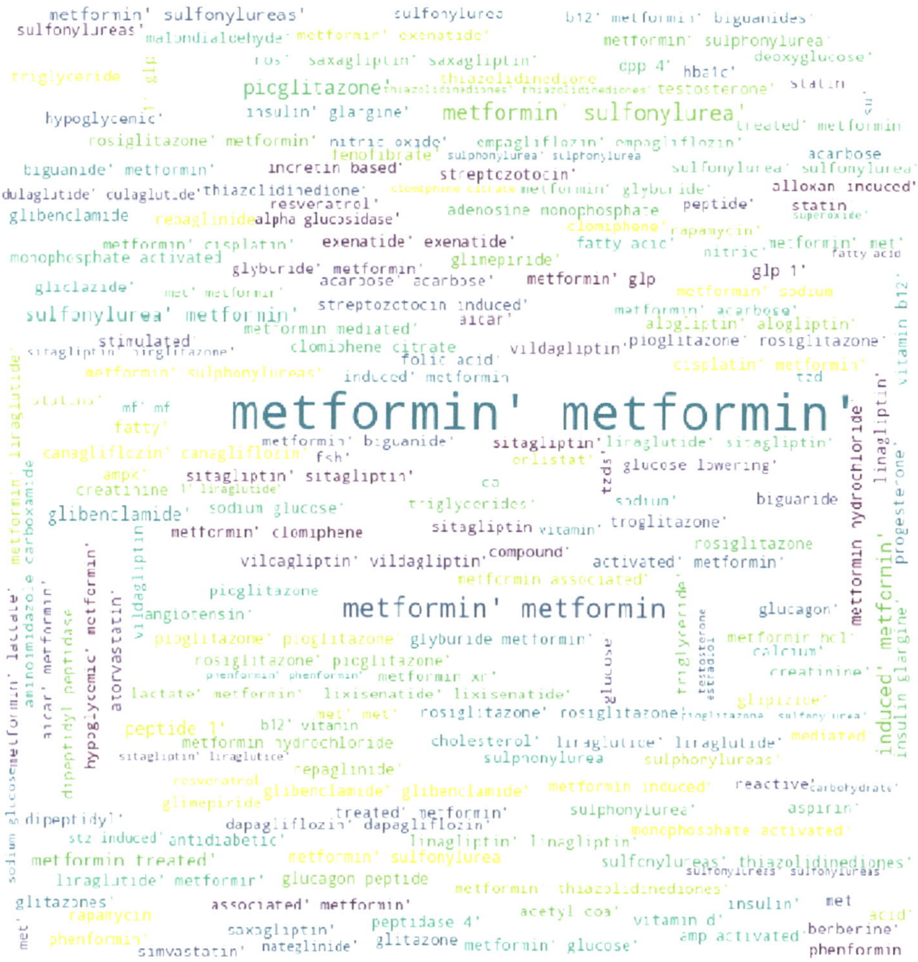

Figure 2.
The word-cloud of the BioBERT model in drugs.

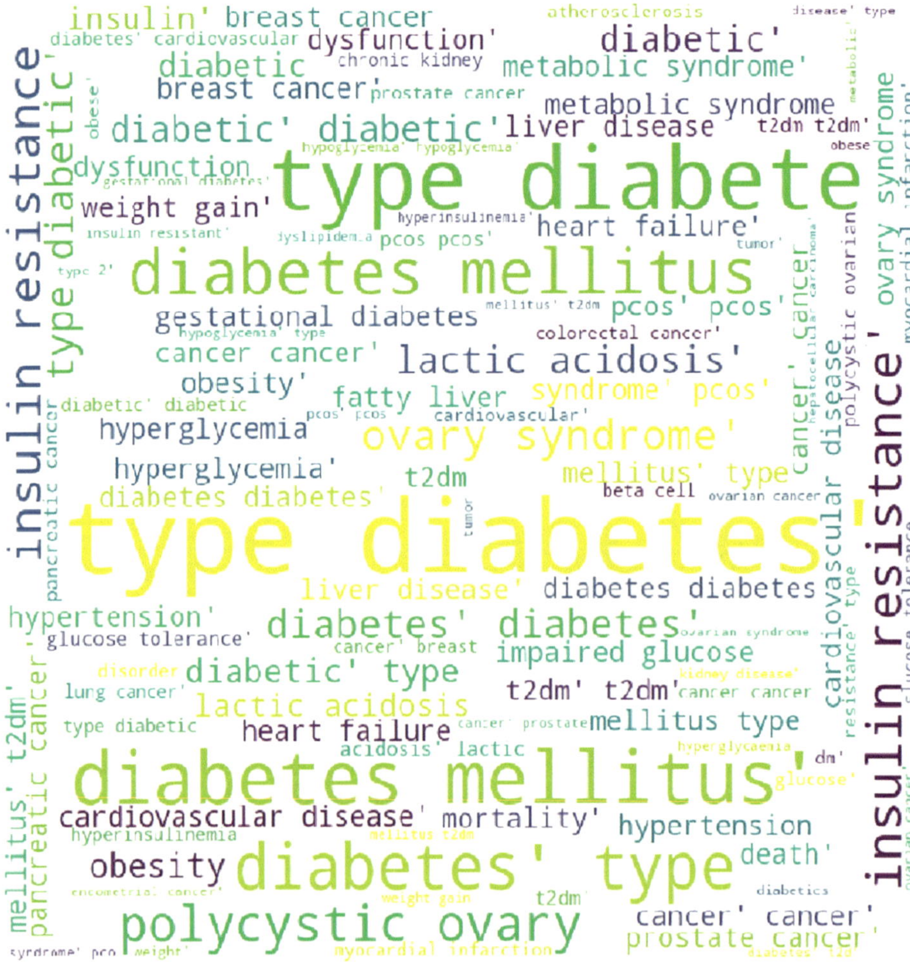

Figure 3.
The word-cloud of the BioBERT model in disease.

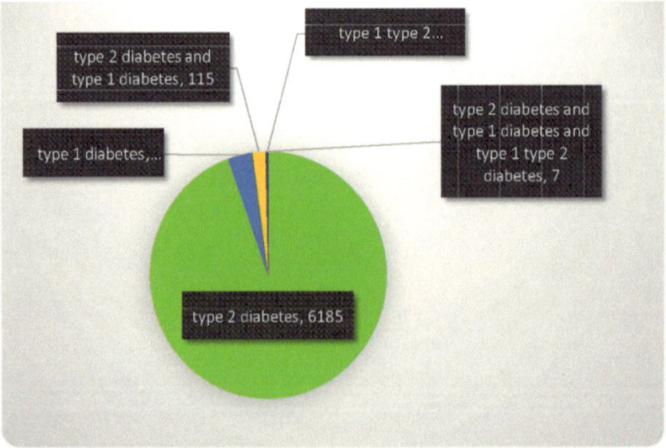

Figure 4.
The word-cloud of the BioBERT model in disease.

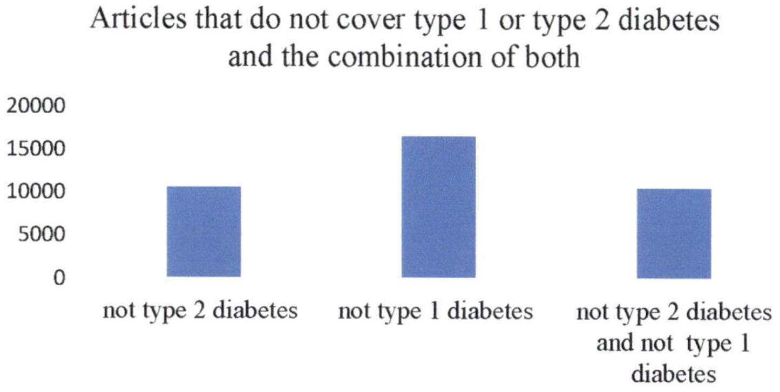

Figure 5.
The word-cloud of the BioBert model in disease.

functions. One of these drug classes is biguanides. Metformin, the only member of this drug group, works in three ways:

- Decreased amount of glucose produced in the liver
- Decreased absorption: the amount of glucose that the body absorbs
- Increased effect of insulin on the body

Diabetes medications are generally prescribed to lower blood glucose For example, in articles, it refers to synthetic alternatives and antidiabetic drugs to reduce perfusion or kidney function, exacerbate the antihypertensive effects, exacerbate metabolic acidosis, and so on (**Figures 3–5**).

According to the NERBIOBERT model, out of 16,781 articles reviewed by the PubMed site and analyzed in the article, 6185 papers refer to type 2 diabetes and 221 papers refer to type 1 diabetes as we know it. Type 2 diabetes is a chronic disease. It is characterized by high levels of sugar in the blood. Type 2 diabetes is also called type 2 diabetes mellitus and adult-onset diabetes. Although, 2388 papers used metformin in type 2 diabetes mellitus, and 1178 articles did not mention any disease at all. Therefore, based on the type of articles, if the adverse use of metformin for the treatment of another disease has been identified, it can be used in the treatment of that disease. What is important in this analysis is a demonstration of the disease and the drug so that by analyzing a large volume of authoritative articles, the use of the approved drug can be used in the treatment of other diseases.

5. Conclusion

Experimental results on the drugs and disease with using advanced deep learning models like Bret show that integrating pretrained biomedical language representation models (i.e. BERT and BioBERT) into a pipe of information extraction methods with multitask learning can improve the ability to collect drug repurposing knowledge from PubMed.

Hitherto, there has not been any clear answer for that in clinical trial, and also, the role of metformin on treatment or prevention of disease remains hypothetical on next step, and we will extract the association between diabetes and other relevant disease with respect to administration of metformin as treatment.

Acknowledgements

The authors have no proprietary, financial, professional, or other personal interest of any nature in any product, service, or company. There is no conflict of interest in this study.

Author details

Zahra Rezaei[1*] and Behnaz Eslami[2]

1 Department of Statistics and Information Technology, Institute of Judiciary, Tehran, Iran

2 Department of Computer Engineering, Science and Research Branch, Islamic Azad University, Tehran, Iran

*Address all correspondence to: z.rezaei2010@gmail.com

References

[1] Dickson M, Gagnon JP. The cost of new drug discovery and development. Discovery Medicine. 2009;**22**(4):172-179

[2] Naylor S, Kauppi MJ, Schonfeld JM. Therapeutic drug repurposing, repositioning and rescue part II: Business review. Drug Discovery World. 2015;**16**:57-72

[3] Liu Z, Fang H, Reagan K, Xu X, Mendrick DL, William Slikker WT Jr. In silico drug repositioning: What we need to know. Drug Discovery Today. 2013;**18**:110-115

[4] Sun P, Guo J, Winnenburg R, Baumbach J. Drug repurposing by integrated literature mining and drug-gene-disease triangulation. Drug Discovery Today. 2017;**22**:615-619

[5] Yang H-T, Ju J-H, Wong Y-T, Shmulevich I, Chiang J H. Literature-based discovery of new candidates for drug repurposing. Briefings in Bioinformatics. 2017;**18**:488-497

[6] Zhu S, Bai Q, Li L, Xu T. Drug repositioning in drug discovery of T2DM and repositioning potential of antidiabetic agents. Computational and Structural Biotechnology Journal. 2022;**20**:2839-2847

[7] Bengio ACPY. Vincent representation learning: A review and new perspectives. IEEE Transactions on Pattern Analysis and Machine Intelligence. 2013;**35**(8):1798-1828

[8] Lee J, Yoon W, Kim S, Kim D, Kim S, So CH, et al. BioBERT: A pre-trained biomedical language representation model for biomedical text mining. Bioinformatics. 2020;**36**(4):1234-1240

[9] Wei C-H, Kao H-Y, Lu Z. PubTator.A web-based text mining tool for assisting biocuration. Nucleic Acids Research. 2013;**41**:W518-W522

[10] Lee S, Kim D, Lee K, Choi J, Kim S, Jeon M, et al. BEST: Next-generation biomedical entity search tool for knowledge discovery from biomedical literature. PLoS One. 2016;**11**(10):e0164680

Section 2

Topical Drug Delivery

Chapter 3

Nanoemulgel: For Promising Topical and Systemic Delivery

Nazneen Sultana, Juber Akhtar, Badruddeen, Mohammad Irfan Khan, Usama Ahmad, Muhammad Arif, Mohammad Ahmad and Tanmay Upadhyay

Abstract

Nanoemulgel delivery system is a fusion of two different delivery systems, wherein the physical state of drug containing nanoemulsion is changed by adding it to the gel matrix, thus enabling more lipophilic drugs to be used in treatment therapies. It solves the major issues such as limiting use of lipophilic drugs, poor oral bioavailability, and unpredictable pharmacokinetic and absorption variations. Simultaneously, its nongreasy nature and easily spreading ability support the patient compliance. Nanoemulgel can be widely used in the treatment of acne, pimple, psoriasis, fungal infection, and inflammation cause by osteoarthritis and rheumatoid arthritis. The delivery of drug via ocular, vaginal, dental, and nose to brain routes for the treatment of diverse local and systemic ailments for instance alopecia, periodontitis, and Parkinson's are possible. In the cosmetic industries, UV absorber nanoemulgel protected skin from sunburn.

Keywords: nanoemulgel, lipophilic, bioavailability, permeability

1. Introduction

Extensive research in the chemical synthetic approaches has led to a huge increment in the poorly water-soluble drug's development [1]. In the present scenario, statistical reports suggest that there are approximately 70% of poor water-soluble new chemical entities (NCEs) [2]. These newly developed drugs possess lipophilic characteristic and are challenging to deliver through the oral route. They have poor oral bioavailability, show variation in intra- as well as intersubject pharmacokinetics, have poor dose proportionality, and have erratic absorption [3]. Researchers have made many strategies to overcome the limitation of poor solubility and bioavailability. Different delivery system formulation development and chemical and/or physical modification of drug moiety can be used to solve the poor solubility issue of drugs. Though there are many drug delivery system approaches, lipid-based drug delivery system has gained much interest in lipophilic drug delivery. It includes macroemulsion, nanoemulsion, niosomes, self-emulsifying formulation, liposomes, solid-lipid nanoparticle, etc. Among all these formulation approaches, emulsion-based preparation can be considered an industrially feasible approach to overcome the limitation of poor bioavailability [4]. Nanoemulsion is capable of improving the topical drug absorption thereby increasing the bioavailability and permeability of lipophilic drug; thus, it can be a good alternative option for drug delivery [5]. Nanoemulsion is further incorporated into gel matrix to prepare nanoemulgel which has even better permeation and stability. So far, there is no review article reported on the promising future of nanoemulgel applications as a delivery system in the treatment of various diseases. This article is a complete package of nanoemulgel comprising information of potent selected formulation component, formulation procedure, advantages over other delivery system, and widespread possible application of nanoemulgel in the treatment therapy. In this article, we have mentioned only reported applications, and there are many to still go in the upcoming future.

Though oral route offers better patient compliance, it has various limitations like gastric irritation, unavoidable side effects, systemic toxicity, and hepatic first-pass metabolism [6]. To avoid all these issues, a nonirritating, non-painful, and a noninvasive topical drug delivery system can be a suitable alternative. It has several advantages over oral route such as targeted site-specific delivery of drug with least systemic toxicity, no gastric irritation, first-pass metabolism bypass, and improved bioavailability of a drug [7, 8]. Apart from many advantages, traditional topical formulations, namely lotions, creams, and ointments suffer from sticky nature, stability issue, low spreadability, etc. which affect the patient's compliance. Whereas, modern transdermal preparations like transparent gel, nanogel, and (micro/nano) emulgel not only have shown improved patient compliance but also improves the formulation efficacy, stability, and safety. Several studies have reported that topical drug delivery system improves the bioavailability of the drug [9, 10]. Bioavailability of lacidipine given through transdermal route was found to be increased by 3.5-fold than the oral route. It may be due to the avoidance of the first-pass metabolism of the drug [9]. In another study conducted by Bhaskar and team, it was found that the topical nanoemulsion of flurbiprofen exhibits 4.4 times more bioavailability than oral delivery [10]. Thus, the bioavailability of a lipophilic drug can be enhanced by the topical drug delivery system. Topical delivery not only reduces the drug metabolism but also improves the permeation across the skin by maintaining longer steady-state delivery of the drug [9].

2. Emulsion-based nano-carrier in topical application

Delivery of a lipophilic drug is a big obstacle for the conventional transdermal delivery system due to low therapeutic potential and poor skin permeability capability. Researches propose that nanoscale-sized transdermal preparation can increase the drug permeability by disrupting the skin bilayer of lipid [11] and extending the drug retention time at the site of action [12, 13]. Nanoemulsion can be a promising carrier delivery of hydrophobic drug, since it has greater thermodynamic stability and higher capability of drug solubilization over emulsion and other dispersion systems. It also has longer shelf life and requires a small amount of external energy for manufacturing [14]. Nanoemulsion is a dispersed system which consists of nanoscale-sized (20–200 nm diameter) droplets solvent composed of an oil phase and water phase and stabilized by the suitable surfactant. Drug is entrapped in the core which is surrounded by emulsifier layer as shown in **Figure 1**. Generally, permeation enhancers are not required when nanoemulsion is used as a carrier for delivery of the lipophilic

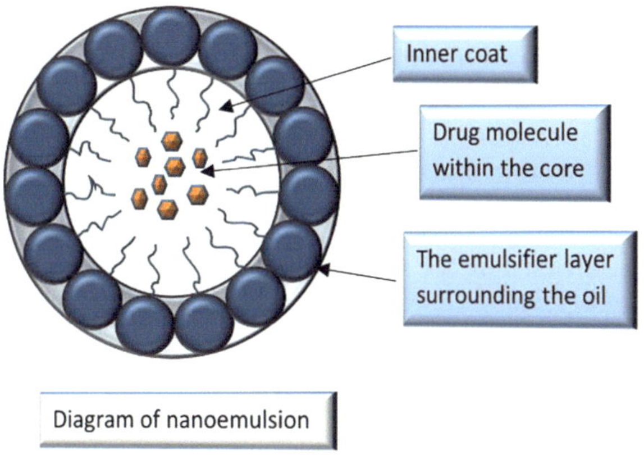

Figure 1.
Structure of nanoemulsion.

drug [15]. It has less tendency of phase separation than other ordinary emulsions which makes it more stable [16]. Different studies have reported better permeation of drug into the skin through nanoemulsion delivery system than conventional ointment [17], cream [18], gel [19], and emulsion [20]. Depending on the type of nanoemulsion, viz. oil-in-water or water-in-oil, it can solubilize both hydrophobic and hydrophilic drug in its structure [21].

In spite of lots of advantages, nanoemulsion suffers from low spreadability, low viscosity, and poor skin retention issue [22]. Due to these, the clinical application of topical nanoemulsion is restrained [23]. Researchers converted nanoemulsion into nanoemulgel by incorporating it into the gel matrix and solved this problem.

2.1 Nanoemulgel as topical drug delivery system

Nanoemulgel is the fusion of two systems: nanoemulsion system and hydrogel system. Both the systems have some limitations, such as nanoemulsion that suffers low spreadability and poor retention, whereas hydrogels are incapable of incorporating lipophilic molecule [24, 25]. Nanoemulgel has different types of polymeric materials, surfactants, and fatty substances of natural, synthetic, and semisynthetic nature with a droplet size range from 5 to 500 nm [26]. Nanoemulgel has the capability to overcome the limitation of both the systems. The lipophilic drug is dissolved in the oil phase of nanoemulsion which is then added to hydrogel base to form nanoemulgel [27] which enables the incorporation of lipophilic drug into a hydrogel, simultaneously improving the viscosity of nanoemulsion. In transdermal drug delivery, nanoemulgel acts as a reservoir of the drug. The drug is first to release from the inner phase to the outer phase and from there into the skin surface. When applied on skin, oily droplets were released from the gel matrix of nanoemulgel, which then penetrate deep into the skin via stratum corneum, and there they directly deliver the drug moiety [23]. The mechanism of drug release depends on the crosslink density as well as the composition of a network of polymer chains [28].

2.2 Potent components for nanoemulgel formulation

Nanoemulgel is a fusion of two separate systems, viz. the nanoemulsion and a gel system. Nanoemulsion acting as a vehicle for drug delivery can be either water-in-oil or oil-in-water type. In both cases, it consists of an oil phase, aqueous phase, surfactant, and sometime cosurfactant. Overview of commonly used major components of nanoemulgel formulation has been apprehended in this section (**Figure 2**).

2.2.1 Oils

Oil is an important component of the nanoemulgel formulation that should be selected appropriately based on the solubility, stability, permeability, and viscosity of the formulation. Vegetable oils/edible oils are not frequently used in nanoemulgel formulation, since they had shown poor emulsification properties and drug solubility [29–31]. Thus, chemically modified oils such as mono or diglyceride or medium-chain triglycerides are commonly used as an oil phase in the nanoemulgel formulation for lipophilic drug delivery [15]. A medium-chain triglyceride, Labrafac, has been used by Syamala and his group to prepare butenafine nanoemulgel [32]. Capryol 90 is another example used as an oil phase in the preparation of nanoemulsion, which has shown better stability of the nanoemulsion formulation of leflunomide and paclitaxel [3, 33].

On the other hand, scientists are focusing on utilizing the supplementary benefit of natural oil in therapeutic effect. Antimicrobial activity of tea tree oil was combined with an antifungal agent itraconazole for a synergistic effect of nanoemulgel preparation against vaginal candidiasis [34]. Another nanoemulgel of curcumin has been reported by Jeengar and team with emu oil. Emu oil obtained from emu bird has analgesic, antipruritic, anesthetic, antioxidants, and anti-inflammatory properties, and it has shown the improvement in permeability of drug in the treatment of joint synovial [35]. Various oils used by different researchers in nanoemulgel preparation are listed in **Table 1**.

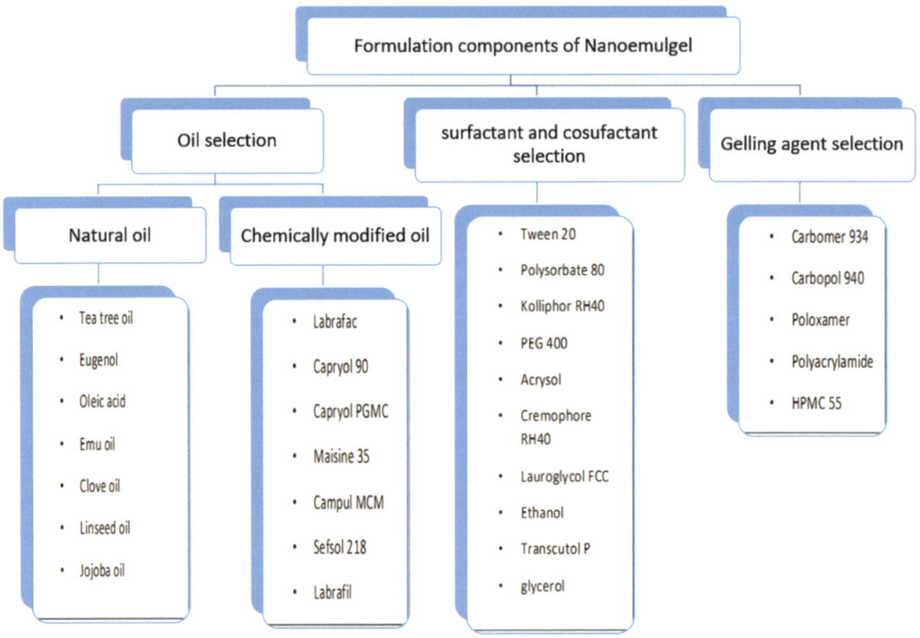

Figure 2.
Potent formulation component of nanoemulgel.

Active Drug	**Oil**	**Surfactant**	**Cosurfactant**	**Gelling agents**	**Reference**
Thymol	Caprylic acid, isopropyl myristate, and tea tree oil	Tween 20	PEG 400	Carbopol 940	[36]
Curcumin	Emu oil	Cremophor RH40	Labrafil M2125CS	Carbopol	[35]
Flurbiprofen	Linseed oil, isopropyl myristate and triacetin	Tween 80	Ethanol + PEG 400 + propylene glycol	Carbopol 940	[37]
Ketoconazole	Labrafac™ LipophileWL1349	Tween 80	PEG 400	Carbopol	[38]
Cyclosporine	Oleic acid	Tween 80	Transcutol P	Guar gum	[24]
Ferulic acid	Isosteryl isostearate	Labrasol	Plurol isostearique	Carbopol 940	[39]
Ropinirole	Capryol 90	Tween 20	Carbitol	Carbopol 934	[15]
Butenafine	Labrafac	Cremophore RH40	Ethanol	Carbopol	[32]
Ketoprofen	Oleic acid	Tween 80	Transcutol P	Carbopol 940	[40]
Piroxicam	Oleic acid	Tween 80	Ethanol	Carbopol 934	[41]
Amphotericin B	Sefsol-218	Tween 80	Transcutol-P	Carbopol	[42]
Aceclofenac and capsaicin	Olive oil and miglyol	Polysorbate 80	Transcutol	Propylene glycol	[43]
Terbinafine hydrochloride	Liquid paraffin	Polysorbate 80	Glycerin	Carbopol 940	[44]
Glibenclamide	Labrafac and triacetin	Tween 80	Diethylene glycol monorthyl ether	Carbopol 934	[45]
Carvedilol	Oleic acid and IPM	Tween 20	Carbitol	Carbopol 934	[46]
Telmisartan	Labrafil	Acrysol	Carbitol	Carbopol	[47]

Table 1.
Various components used in different nanoemulgel formulations.

2.2.2 Surfactant and cosurfactant

Surfactant reduces the interfacial tension between the mixtures of two immiscible liquids and changes the dispersion entropy, thus stabilizing thermodynamically unstable emulsion system. Selection of appropriate surfactant for nanoemulgel is based on the safety, stability, high drug loading capacity as well as good emulsification properties [31]. Also, the surfactant should be selected based on the solubility with oil like Tween 20 that was used on the basis of solubility of Capryol 90 and oleic acid [15, 40].

Cosurfactant may combine with surfactant and help in the emulsification process by disrupting the interfacial film. It may also help in solubilization of oil [15].

Depending on the physicochemical properties, most frequently used cosurfactants in nanoemulsion and nanoemulgel preparation are propylene glycol, PEG 400, ethanol, transcutol P, carbitol, etc. [35, 40]. Studies suggest that with the increase in the concentration of cosurfactant, the area of nanoemulsion in phase diagram decreases [48, 49].

2.2.3 Aqueous solvents

Aqueous solvents act as the aqueous phase in emulsion preparation. Worldwide widely used aqueous solvents are ethanol and water.

2.2.4 Gelling agents

Carbapol 934, Carbapol 940, and hydroxy propyl methyl cellulose (HPMC) are widely used gelling agent for nanoemulgel. They increased the thickness of the formulation and may interact with the surfactant to modify the viscosity of the formulation [41]. It is added to the nanoemulsion preparation to change the physical state of nanoemulsion formulation from liquid to gel, thus solving the problem of low spreadability, low viscosity, and poor skin retention issue of nanoemulsion.

2.2.5 Miscellaneous components

To protect the formulation from microbial attack and increase the shelf life of formulation, preservatives are added in the preparation. Most commonly used preservatives are methylparaben, benzoic acid, propylparaben, benzalkonium chloride, etc. Antioxidants like butylate hydroxyl toluene, butylate hydroxyl anisole, and ascorbyl palmitate are used to prevent oxidative degradation of formulation components and to prevent loss of moisture, glycerin and propylene glycol are used as humectants [50]. Hence, the stability of the nanoemulsion and nanoemulgel preparation increased.

2.3 Preparation of nanoemulgel formulation

Two steps are involved in the manufacturing of nanoemulgel. The first step is nanoemulsion formulation which is then incorporated into a gelling agent in the second step to form nanoemulgel. **Figure 3** schematically represents the procedure of preparation of nanoemulgel.

Methods used for the preparation of nanoemulsion can be high-energy emulsification methods or low-energy emulsification methods [49, 51]. In high-energy emulsification methods, external energy is applied which rupture the oil phase to form nanosized droplets in the aqueous phase. It includes ultrasonic emulsification and high-pressure homogenization. Solvent displacement method, phase inversion composition method, and phase inversion temperature method are low-energy emulsification in which low energy is required for prepared nanoemulsion [21].

2.3.1 Procedure for nanoemulsion preparation

The selected surfactant is dissolved in either the aqueous phase or the oil phase. Based on the solubility, the drug is then added and solubilized in the oil phase or

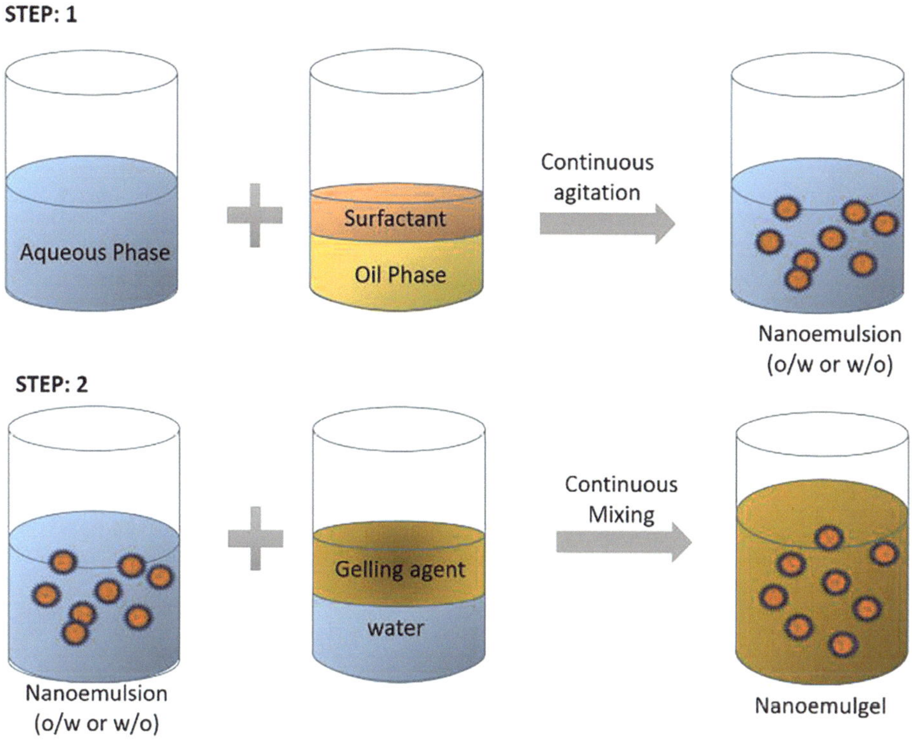

Figure 3.
Procedure of nanoemulgel preparation.

aqueous phase followed by heating. Then one phase is gradually added into another with continuous stirring till the temperature of the mixture reaches to room temperature.

2.3.2 Procedure for nanoemulgel preparation

The appropriate gelling agent is dissolved in distilled water with continuous stirring to prepare gel base. The pH of prepared gel is adjusted, then the nanoemulsion system is incorporated slowly into the prepared gel at a particular ratio with continuous stirring to get nanoemulgel preparation.

2.4 Advantages of nanoemulgel

Nanoemulgel preparations have various advantages over other topical as well as conventional preparation. Some of the advantages are listed as follows (**Figure 4**).

2.4.1 Incorporation of lipophilic drug

The lipophilic drug moieties base show improper drug release mechanism in the gel due to its insolubility in aqueous base. Fusion of the hydrogel system with emulsion system enables the incorporation of lipophilic drug into the aqueous base, thus improving the release mechanism of the drug. Lipophilic drug is dissolved in the oil phase of emulsion which is then incorporated into hydrogel system [52].

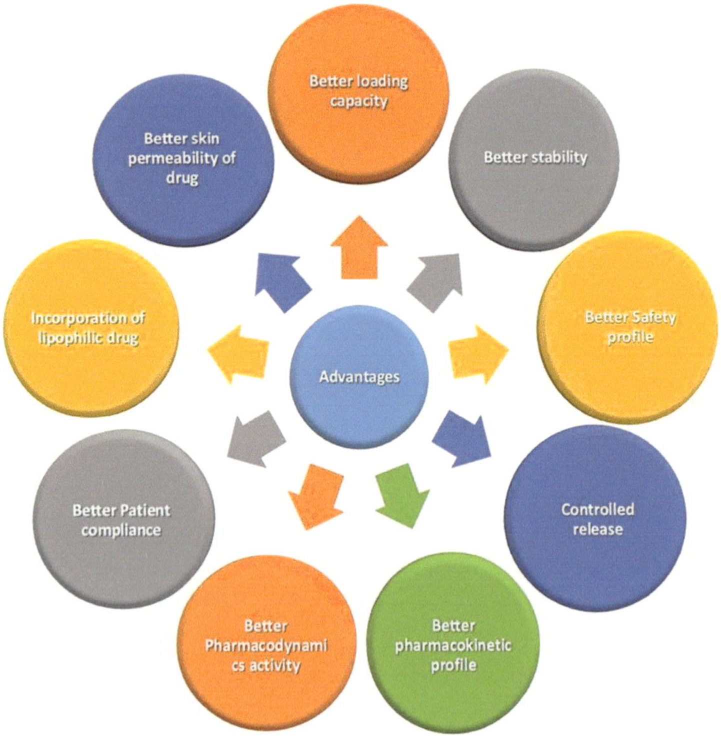

Figure 4.
Advantages of nanoemulgel preparation.

2.4.2 Better loading capacity

Better loading capacity has been observed by nanoemulgel as compared to than other novel drug delivery systems. Due to its nanoscale size, it has a larger surface area and better entrapment efficiency which enable it to load more amount of drugs in its network-like system [52].

2.4.3 Better stability

Nanoemulgel system is more stable than other transdermal drug delivery system, because it decreases the interfacial as well as the surface tension of the formulation, which make it superior from a conventional transdermal delivery system [53].

2.4.4 Controlled release

Nanoemulgel acts as a drug reservoir and has shown prolong residence time leading to sustain release of the drug. Thus, it is beneficial for the drugs having shorter half-life [52].

2.4.5 Better pharmacokinetic profile

Nanoemulgel formulation gives higher T_{max} and peak plasma concentration of lipophilic drugs than the conventional gel as well as oral formulation. Thereby, nanoemulgel preparation improves the bioavailability of lipophilic drug many folds than the other lipophilic drug formulations [53].

2.4.6 Better pharmacodynamics activity

Improved permeability of nanoemulgel preparation through the skin enables more drugs to penetrate into the site of action. This enhances the pharmacodynamic activity of the drug increasing its therapeutic efficacy.

2.4.7 Better patient compliance

Major issue with the transdermal preparation is the sticky nature and low spreading coefficient which require rubbing mechanism. Nanoemulgel being nonsticky and easily spreadable preparation results in better patient compliance than other transdermal preparations [28].

2.4.8 Enhanced drug permeability through skin

Nanoemulgel has shown significant enhancement in the permeability of the drug through skin than other formulation since from nanoemulgel preparation, the drug can permeate the skin layer through both paracellular and transcellular route, whereas, in nanoemulsion, only transcellular permeation route is seen [53]. Comparison of cumulative drug permeability through the skin from different formulation is represented in **Figure 5** [24].

2.4.9 Better safety profile

Nanoemulgel bypasses the first-pass metabolism, thus solving one of the major problems of drug, that is, the oral side effect. It does not cause skin irritation or any toxicity on the application [53].

3. Health claim

A significant number of the nanoemulgel formulation of drugs has been carried out and reported by various researchers to show its application as a more potent and effective drug delivery system. Some of the studies have shown outstanding result over the conventional oral drug delivery system, suggesting a promising future of nanoemulgel application.

3.1 Acne and pimple

Thymol nanoemulgel formulation for acne vulgaris, a common chronic skin disease, was prepared by Ahmad and team. The preparation showed better efficacy [36].

3.2 Psoriasis

It is the skin condition in which skin cells build up and form itchy, dry patches, and scales. A nanoemulgel formulation of leflunomide by Pund and team showed considerably higher anti-psoriatic and anti-melanoma activity in human keratinocyte

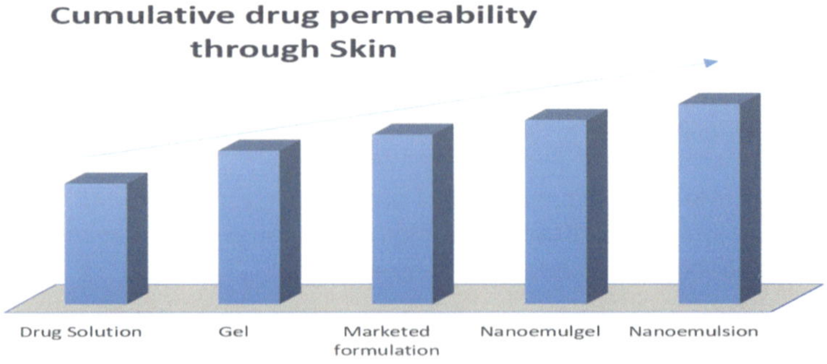

Figure 5.
Comparative representation of cumulative cyclosporine permeated through the skin of albino rat from different formulations. Regenerated from [24].

cell line due to improved permeability of drug. Amount of drug deposited in the skin after 12 hours by nanoemulgel was found to be sixfold more than ordinary gel [33]. In another study by Somagoni and team, nanoemulgel showed 3.22- and 2.01-fold more reduction of ear swelling than drug solution and marketed product, respectively, in psoriatic-like model [43].

3.3 Fungal infection

High skin permeability of nanoemulgel has made it a better alternative for the faster treatment of fungal infection. Syamala has reported that it took only 12 days to Butenafine nanoemulgel to cure fungus-infected rat skin, whereas cream took 16 days [32]. Nanoemulgel has also shown a notable increase in antifungal activity of the drug. Higher area of inhibition zone was observed with Ketoconazole nanoemulgel than drug solution when incubated for 48 hours [38]. Nanoemulgel of Amphotericin B can overcome formulation limitation of Amphotericin B making it a better alternative to painful intravenous administration. It could be used as a stable, effective, and safe carrier for sustained and enhanced localized delivery of Amphotericin B against fungal infection [42].

3.4 Inflammation and pain due to osteoarthritis and rheumatic arthritis

Nanoemulgel is a better alternative for poor water-soluble anti-inflammatory drugs, and it also bypasses the related oral side effects of drugs like gastrointestinal irritation, renal, and cardiovascular problems, etc. Many researchers have reported remarkably higher activity of anti-inflammatory drugs in nanoemulgel formulation than other drug carrier system [35, 40, 54–57]. Nanoemulgel of ketoprofen, an extensively utilized non steroidal anti inflammatory drugs (NSAIDs) for rheumatoid arthritis and osteoarthritis treatment, was developed by Arora and team. Along with enhancing the skin permeability and solubility of ketoprofen, it also bypasses the problems related to chronic oral delivery of ketoprofen. Comparison of the optimized formulation with the marketed product and drug solution showed 1.5- and 2-fold higher permeability, respectively [40].

Another common drug used in osteoarthritis and rheumatoid arthritis is piroxicam. It is also used in the treatment of the musculoskeletal and joint disorder. It also possesses the problem of poor solubility along with undesirable side effect on stomach and kidney. Dhawan and team reported that piroxicam nanoemulgel can be used as a feasible alternative [41].

Apart from these, attempt has also made to establish the stability, efficacy, and safety of certain drugs with anti-inflammatory activity which has poor solubility and permeability profile and/or oral side effect like curcumin [35], Swietenia macrophylla [27], Lornoxicam [54], Nimesulide [55], mangosteen [56], and diclofenac diethylamine [57]. **Figure 6** represents the comparison of anti-inflammatory effect of flurbiprofen nanoemulgel by Radhika and Guruprasad with marketed preparation [37].

3.5 Periodontal disease

Dental nanoemulgel preparation is intended for periodontal delivery of drug to treat chronic bacterial infection of the gum and bone supporting teeth. Periodontal disease causes inflammation of gum forming pockets which may lead to gum tissue and bone damage. Srivastava and team formulated syringeable ketoprofen nanoemulgel for intra-pocket delivery and found satisfied pharmaceutical characterization offering sustained release of ketoprofen into the pocket. Significant reduction was observed in alveolar bone loss, gingival index, and tooth motility by ketoprofen nanoemulgel due to decreased cytokine levels [58]. Whereas, the study of Nayak and team suggested that controlled released delivery of Quercetin nanoemulgel can be used successfully in periodontitis [59].

3.6 Corneal fungus infection

Ocular nanoemulgel can be better alternative drug delivery system to the conventional eye drops to cure corneal fungal infection. Permeation of fluconazole from nanoemulgel preparation was found four times that of commercial fluconazole eye drop due to high permeation, sustained release of drug, and prolongation in the pre-corneal residence time. Prolong release was achieved by in situ gelation of Gellan gum due to its crosslinking with tear fluid. Fluconazole nanoemulgel formulation showed no sign of any ocular irritation and tissue damage [60]. Whereas, Tayel used a rabbit model to successfully control the release rate of terbinafine-HCL nanoemulgel, which can be an effective alternative to conventional eye drop for ocular fungal infection, into the rabbit aqueous humor [61].

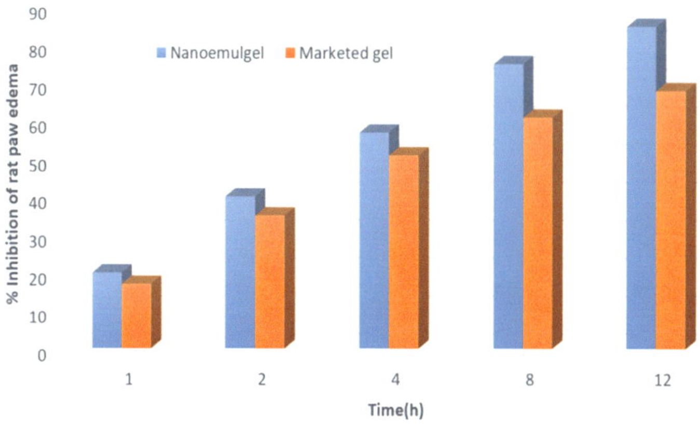

Figure 6.
Graphical representation of improvement in anti-inflammatory effect of nanoemulgel of flurbiprofen. Regenerated from [56].

3.7 Vaginal candidiasis

A thermo-sensitive nanoemulgel of itraconazole with tea tree oil was prepared for patients suffering from periodic vaginal candidiasis. Antimicrobial activity of itraconazole and tea tree oil combined to give synergistic effect covering cure for wide range microbial infection [34].

3.8 Alopecia

Minoxidil is the commonly used drug for the treatment of hair loss also known as alopecia. Nanoemulgel is capable of increasing solubility and permeability of drug through the skin; hence, nanoemulgel preparation of minoxidil will be more effective and safer than conventional preparation present in the market for the treatment of alopecia areata [62].

3.9 Insomnia

Nasal nanoemulgel of zaleplon was formulated by Hosny and Banjar for the treatment of insomnia. The main objective was to solve the problem with marketed zaleplon tablet. Zaleplon tablet suffers from poor bioavailability due to extensive first-pass metabolism and delayed onset of action due to poor aqueous solubility. Nasal zaleplon nanoemulgel showed eight times more bioavailability than the marketed zaleplon tablet [63].

3.10 Parkinson's disease

Selegiline HCL-loaded nanoemulgel possess better sustains release effect of the drug and higher bioavailability than the conventional gel and a marketed tablet. Bioavailability was reported to be 5.53 and 6.56 times that of normal gel and tablet [64].

Product brand name	Active pharmaceutical ingredient(s)	Manufacturers	Application
Benzolait AZ emulgel	Benzoylperoxide	Roydermal	Pimple and blacks on skin
Coolnac Gel emulgel 1%	Diclofenac diethyl ammonium	Chumchon	Inflammation and pain due to trauma
Diclobar emulgel	Diclofenac diethyl amine	Barakat Pharma	Inflammation due to trauma and rheumatic diseases
Levorage emulgel	Liquorice, hibiscus, and natural extract	THD Ltd	Anal fissures
Meloxic emulgel	Meloxicum	Laboratories Provet	Musculoskeletal pain management and inflammation
Miconaz-H-emulgel	Miconazole nitrate, hydrocortisone	Medical Union Pharmaceutics	Skin infection by candida
Reumadep emulgel	Ashwagandha, myrrh, arnica, rosemary, mint, and cloves	Erbozeta	Inflammation and pain due to trauma
Voltaren emulgel	Diclofenac diethyl ammonium	Novartis Pharma	Osteoarthritis joint pain
Voveron emulgel	Diclofenac diethyl amine	Novartis Pharma	Osteoarthritis joint pain

Table 2.
Available marketed emulgel preparations.

Microemulgel loaded with rotigotine has also shown significantly higher bioavailability than marketed patch of rotigotine in the treatment of Parkinson's disease [65].

3.11 Cosmetics

Use of nanotechnology in cosmetics is very common. Fullerenes, solid-lipid nanoparticle, liposomes, nanosomes, etc., are already nourishing in cosmetic industries. Ferulic acid nanoemulgel was developed by Harwansh and team to protect the skin damage from harmful UV radiation. Ferulic acid strongly absorbs the UV radiation. Its incorporation into nanoemulgel system made it effective for more than 4 hours on the UV-exposed skin [39].

Currently available marketed emulgel products for the treatment of acne and pimple, inflammation, and pain caused by osteoarthritis and rheumatoid arthritis and skin infection have been listed in **Table 2**.

4. Mechanism involved to enhance permeability and bioavailability from nanoemulgel preparations

The skin permeability as well as bioavailability of nanoemulgel may be enhanced by various mechanisms. Some of the studied mechanisms with types of nanoemulgel are listed in **Table 3**.

Types of nanoemulgel	Mechanism of permeability/bioavailability	References
Conjugate of curcumin	Induced apoptosis in cancer cells, suppressing the expression of NF-κB, TNF-α, and COX-2 cellular targets	[66]
Clove essential oil	Dispersion of the nanoemulsion in the polymeric matrices of the prepared nanoemulgel	[67]
Snakehead fish (pphiocephalus striatus)	Ex vivo transdermal permeation value	[68]
Methotrexate	Change in temperature experienced by the nanogel	[69]
Terbinafine	Ex vivo drug permeation and in vivo antifungal activity	[70]
Paclitaxel	Nanogel exerts high cytotoxicity to cancer cells and reverses multidrug resistance effectively	[71]
Diphenhydramine	First-order kinetics and Fickian diffusion	[72]
Raloxifene hydrochloride	Ex vivo permeation, histopathology, SEM, DSC, and CLSM studies	[73]
Desonide	DES, Franz diffusion cell system, CLSM	[74]
Ketoconazole	Ex vivo permeation	[75]
Telmisartan	Ex vivo permeation, first-order reaction, and Higuchi model with non-Fickian diffusion	[76]
Ibuprofen	Drug diffusion, however, drug partition, and matrix erosion	[77]
Piroxicam	Franz diffusion cell	[78]

NF: nuclear factor, TNF: tumor necrosis factor, SEM: scanning electron microscopy, DSC: differential scan calorimetry, DES: dielectric spectroscopy, CLSM: confocal laser scanning microscopy.

Table 3.
Mechanism involved in enhancing permeability and bioavailability of some nanoemulgel preparations.

5. Conclusion

Nanoemulgel has been found to be extraordinarily good vehicle system for hydrophobic drug delivery. High drug loading due to better solubilizing efficacy, improved bioavailability due to better permeability, and capability to control the release of drug make it a potent alternative delivery system in the treatment of various diseases. Application of nanoemulgel preparation in the treatment of acne, pimple, psoriasis, fungal infection, and inflammation due to osteoarthritis as well as rheumatoid arthritis has shown significantly higher efficacy. Besides transdermal application, it can also be applied for ocular, vaginal, dental, and nose to brain delivery of drug for the treatment of diverse local and systemic ailments such as alopecia, periodontitis, and Parkinson's disease. Nanoemulgel has also shown its application in the cosmetic industries as a UV absorber nanoemulgel to protect skin from sunburn. Precisely, the nanoemulgel system has a marvelous ability to be applied in various local and systemic ailments. Some preparations are already present in the market, whereas others need a further clinical study to launch the product in the market.

Author details

Nazneen Sultana, Juber Akhtar*, Badruddeen, Mohammad Irfan Khan, Usama Ahmad, Muhammad Arif, Mohammad Ahmad and Tanmay Upadhyay
Faculty of Pharmacy, Integral University, Lucknow, India

*Address all correspondence to: jakhtar@iul.ac.in

References

[1] Weissig V, Lizano C, Torchilin VP. Selective DNA release from DQAsome/DNA complexes at mitochondria-like membranes. Drug Delivery. 2000;7:1-5. DOI: 10.1080/107175400266722

[2] Beig A, Miller JM, Lindley D, Carr RA, Zocharski P, Agbaria R, et al. Head-to-head comparison of different solubility-enabling formulations of etoposide and their consequent solubility-permeability interplay. Journal of Pharmaceutical Sciences. 2015;**104**:2941-2947. DOI: 10.1002/jps.24496

[3] Choudhury H, Gorain B, Karmakar S, Biswas E, Dey G, Barik R, et al. Improvement of cellular uptake, *in vitro* antitumor activity and sustained release profile with increased bioavailability from a nanoemulsion platform. International Journal of Pharmaceutics. 2014;**460**:131-143. DOI: 10.1016/j.ijpharm.2013.10.055

[4] Wadhwa J, Nair A, Kumria R. Emulsion forming drug delivery system for lipophilic drugs. Acta Poloniae – Drug Research. 2012;**69**:179-191

[5] Abolmaali SS, Tamaddon AM, Farvadi FS, Daneshamuz S, Moghimi H. Pharmaceutical nanoemulsions and their potential topical and transdermal applications. Iranian Journal of Pharmaceutical Sciences. 2011;**7**:139-150

[6] Kotta S, Khan AW, Ansari SH, Sharma RK, Ali J. Anti HIV nanoemulsion formulation: Optimization and *in vitro-in vivo* evaluation. International Journal of Pharmaceutics. 2014;**462**:129-134. DOI: 10.1016/j.ijpharm.2013.12.038

[7] Ali J, Baboota S, Iqbal MA, Sahni JK, Md S, Dang S. Nanostructured lipid carriers system: Recent advances in drug delivery. Journal of Drug Targeting. 2012;**20**:813-830. DOI: 10.3109/1061186x.2012.716845

[8] Kaur J, Kaur J, Jaiswal S, Gupta G. Recent advances in topical drug delivery system. Pharmaceutical Research. 2016;**6**(7):6353-6369

[9] Gannu R, Palem CR, Yamsani VV, Yamsani SK, Yamsani MR. Enhanced bioavailability of lacidipine via microemulsion based transdermal gels: Formulation optimization, *ex vivo* and *in vivo* characterization. International Journal of Pharmaceutics. 2010;**388**:231-241. DOI: 10.1016/j.ijpharm.2009.12.050

[10] Bhaskar K, Anbu J, Ravichandiran V, Venkateswarlu V, Rao YM. Lipid nanoparticles for transdermal delivery of flurbiprofen: Formulation, in vitro, ex vivo and in vivo studies. Lipids in Health and Disease. 2009;**8**:1-15. DOI: 10.1186/1476-511X-8-6

[11] Shakeel F, Baboota S, Ahuja A, Ali J, Shafiq S. Skin permeation mechanism and bioavailability enhancement of celecoxib from transdermally applied nanoemulsion. Journal of Nanobiotechnology. 2008;**6**:1-11. DOI: 10.1186/1477-3155-6-8

[12] Huang X, Peng X, Wang Y, Wang Y, Shin DM, El-Sayed MA, et al. A reexamination of active and passive tumor targeting by using rod-shaped gold nanocrystals and covalently conjugated peptide ligands. ACS Nano. 2010;**4**:5887-5896. DOI: 10.1021/nn102055s

[13] Delouise LA. Applications of nanotechnology in dermatology. Journal of Investigative Dermatology.

2012;**132**:964-975. DOI: 10.1038/jid.2011.425

[14] Muller RH, Benita S, Bohm B, editors. Emulsions and Nanosuspensions for the Formulation of Poorly Soluble Drugs. Vol. 8. Stuttgart: Medpharm Scientific Publishers; 1998. pp. 149-173. DOI: 10.1208/pt0802028

[15] Rizwan M, Azeem A, Aqil M, Talegaonkar S, Khar RK, Ahmad FJ, et al. Nanoemulsion components screening and selection: A technical note. AAPS PharmSciTech. 2009;**10**:69-76. DOI: 10.1208/s12249-008-9178-x

[16] Kim BS, Won M, Lee KM, Kim CS. *In vitro* permeation studies of nanoemulsions containing ketoprofen as a model drug. Drug Delivery. 2008;**15**:465-469. DOI: 10.1080/10717540802328599

[17] De Moraes CAF, Ceschel GC, Bergamante V, Fini A, Ronchi C. Control of transdermal permeation of hydrocortisone acetate from hydrophilic and lipophilic formulations. AAPS PharmSciTech. 2008;**9**:762-768. DOI: 10.1208/s12249-008-9107-z

[18] Teichmann A, Heuschkel S, Jacobi U, Presse G, Neubert RHH, Sterry W, et al. Comparison of stratum corneum penetration and localization of a lipophilic model drug applied in an o/w microemulsion and an amphiphilic cream. European Journal of Pharmaceutics and Biopharmaceutics. 2007;**67**:699-706. DOI: 10.1016/j.ejpb.2007.04.006

[19] Abramović Z, Šuštaršič U, Teskač K, Šentjurc M, Kristl J. Influence of nanosized delivery systems with benzyl nicotinate and penetration enhancers on skin oxygenation. International Journal of Pharmaceutics. 2008;**359**:220-227. DOI: 10.1016/j.ijpharm.2008.03.014

[20] Bolzinger MA, Briançon S, Pelletier J, Fessi H, Chevalier Y. Percutaneous release of caffeine from microemulsion, emulsion and gel dosage forms. European Journal of Pharmaceutics and Biopharmaceutics. 2008;**68**:446-451. DOI: 10.1016/j.ejpb.2007.10.018

[21] Date AA, Desai N, Dixit R, Nagarsenker M. Self-nanoemulsifying drug delivery systems: Formulation insights, applications and advances. Nanomedicine (London). 2010;**5**:1595-1616. DOI: 10.2217/nnm.10.126

[22] Khurana S, Jain NK, Bedi PMS. Nanoemulsion based gel for transdermal delivery of meloxicam: Physico-chemical, mechanistic investigation. Life Science. 2013;**92**:383-392. DOI: 10.1016/j.lfs.2013.01.005

[23] Mou D, Chen H, Du D, Mao C, Wan J, Xu H, et al. Hydrogel-thickened nanoemulsion system for topical delivery of lipophilic drugs. International Journal of Pharmaceutics. 2008;**353**:270-276. DOI: 10.1016/j.ijpharm.2007.11.051

[24] Begur M, Pai VK, Gowda DV, Srivastava A, Raghundan HV, et al. Pelagia Research Library enhanced permeability of cyclosporine from a transdermally applied nanoemulgel. Der Pharmacia Sinica. 2015;**6**:69-79

[25] Guo R, Deng L, Dong A, Zhao F, Zhang J, Yao D. Composites of polymer hydrogels and nanoparticulate systems for biomedical and pharmaceutical applications. Nanomaterials. 2015;**5**:2054-2130. DOI: 10.3390/nano5042054

[26] Anand K, Ray S, Rahman M, Shaharyar A, Bhowmik R, Bera R, et al. Nano-emulgel: Emerging as a smarter topical lipidic emulsion-based nanocarrier for skin healthcare

applications. Recent Patents on Antiinfective Drug Discovery. 2019;**14**:16-35

[27] Eid AM. Preparation, characterization and anti-inflammatory activity of Swietenia macrophylla nanoemulgel. Journal of Nanomedicine & Nanotechnology. 2014;**05**:1-10. DOI: 10.4172/2157-7439.1000190

[28] Chellapa P, Mohamed AT, Keleb EI, Elmahgoubi A, Eid AM, Issa YS, et al. Nanoemulsion and nanoemulgel as a topical formulation. IOSR Journal of Pharmacy. 2015;**5**:43-47 Available from: http://www.iosrphr.org/papers/v5i10/F0510043047.pdf

[29] Aithal GC, Narayan R, Nayak UY. Nanoemulgel: A promising phase in drug delivery. Current Pharmaceutical Design. 2020;**26**:279-291

[30] Warisnoicharoen W, Lansley AB, Lawrence MJ. Nonionic oil-in-water microemulsions: The effect of oil type on phase behaviour. International Journal of Pharmaceutics. 2000;**198**:7-27. DOI: 10.1016/S0378-5173(99)00406-8

[31] Tiwary A, Sood J, Thatai P, Jindal M, Bhandari S, Sapra B. A critical appraisal of microemulsions for drug delivery: Part I. Therapeutic Delivery. 2013;**4**:1547-1564. DOI: 10.4155/tde.13.116

[32] Syamala U. Development & optimization of allyl amine antifungal nanoemulgel using 2 3 factorial design : For the treatment of tinea Pedis. European Scientific Journal. 2013;**4**:597-605

[33] Pund S, Pawar S, Gangurde S, Divate D. Transcutaneous delivery of leflunomide nanoemulgel: Mechanistic investigation into physicomechanical characteristics, *in vitro* anti-psoriatic and anti-melanoma activity. International Journal of Pharmaceutics. 2015;**487**:148-156. DOI: 10.1016/j.ijpharm.2015.04.015

[34] Iqbal Z, Manzoor N, Mirza MA, Mallick MN, Ahmad S, Talegaonkar S. Development of a novel synergistic thermosensitive gel for vaginal candidiasis: An *in vitro*, *in vivo* evaluation. Colloids Surfaces B Biointerfaces. 2012;**103**:275-282. DOI: 10.1016/j.colsurfb.2012.10.038

[35] Jeengar MK, Rompicharla SVK, Shrivastava S, Chella N, Shastri NR, Naidu VGM, et al. Emu oil based nano-emulgel for topical delivery of curcumin. International Journal of Pharmaceutics. 2016;**506**:222-236. DOI: 10.1016/j.ijpharm.2016.04.052

[36] Garg A, Gautam A, Ahmad J, Jain K, Komath S, Bano M. Topical nano-emulgel for skin disorders: Formulation approach and characterization. Recent Patents on Anti-Infective Drug Discovery. 2018;**14**:1-13. DOI: 10.2174/1574891x14666181129115213

[37] Radhika PR, Guruprasad S. Nanoemulsion based emulgel formulation of lipophilic drug for topical delivery. International Journal of PharmTech Research. 2016;**9**:210-223

[38] Mahtab A, Jain GK, Ahmad FJ, Naz Z, Mallick N, Anwar M. Transungual delivery of ketoconazole nanoemulgel for the effective management of onychomycosis. AAPS PharmSciTech. 2016;**17**:1477-1490. DOI: 10.1208/s12249-016-0488-0

[39] Harwansh RK, Mukherjee PK, Bahadur S, Biswas R. Enhanced permeability of ferulic acid loaded nanoemulsion based gel through skin against UVA mediated oxidative stress. Life Sciences. 2015;**141**:202-211. DOI: 10.1016/j.lfs.2015.10.001

[40] Arora R, Aggarwal G, Harikumar SL, Kaur K. Nanoemulsion based hydrogel for enhanced transdermal delivery of ketoprofen. Advances in Pharmacy. 2014;**2014**:1-12. DOI: 10.1155/2014/468456

[41] Aggarwal G, Dhawan B, Harikumar S. Enhanced transdermal permeability of piroxicam through novel nanoemulgel formulation. International Journal of Pharmaceutical Investigation. 2014;**4**:65. DOI: 10.4103/2230-973x.133053

[42] Ahmed FJ, Hussain A, Ahsan MN, Samad A, Singh SK, Haque MW, et al. Nanoemulsion gel-based topical delivery of an antifungal drug: *In vitro* activity and *in vivo* evaluation. Drug Delivery. 2014;**23**:642-657. DOI: 10.3109/10717544.2014.933284

[43] Somagoni J, Patel AR, Boakye CHA, Singh M, Zucolotto V, Mendonca Faria HA, et al. Nanomiemgel - A novel drug delivery system for topical application - *In vitro* and *in vivo* evaluation. PLoS One. 2014;**9**:e115952. DOI: 10.1371/journal.pone.0115952

[44] Karri VVSNR, Raman SK, Kuppusamy G, Mulukutla S, Ramaswamy S, Malayandi R. Terbinafine hydrochloride loaded nanoemulsion based gel for topical application. Journal of Pharmaceutical Investigation. 2015;**45**:79-89. DOI: 10.1007/s40005-014-0149-9

[45] Wais M, Samad A, Nazish I, Khale A, Aqil M, Khan M. Formulation development *ex-vivo* and *in-vivo* evaluation of nanoemulsion. International Journal of Pharmacy and Pharmaceutical Sciences. 2013;**5**:747-754

[46] Singh BP, Kumar B, Jain SK, Shafaat K. Development and characterization of a nanoemulsion gel formulation for transdermal delivery of carvedilol. International Journal of Drug Development & Research. 2012;**4**:151-161

[47] Aparna C, Srinivas P, Patnaik KSKR. Enhanced transdermal permeability of telmisartan by a novel nanoemulsion gel. International Journal of Pharmacy and Pharmaceutical Sciences. 2015;7(4):335-342

[48] Shafiq S, Shakeel F, Talegaonkar S, Ahmad FJ, Khar RK, Ali M. Development and bioavailability assessment of ramipril nanoemulsion formulation. European Journal of Pharmaceutics and Biopharmaceutics. 2007;**66**:227-243. DOI: 10.1016/j.ejpb.2006.10.014

[49] Anton N, Vandamme TF. The universality of low-energy nano-emulsification. International Journal of Pharmaceutics. 2009;**377**:142-147. DOI: 10.1016/j.ijpharm.2009.05.014

[50] Dev A, Chodankar R, Shelke O. Emulgels : A novel topical drug delivery system. Pharmaceutical and Biological Evaluations. 2015;**2**:64-75

[51] Singh H, Flanagan J, Rades T, Neil Pinder D, Kortegaard K. Solubilisation of soybean oil in microemulsions using various surfactants. Food Hydrocolloids. 2005;**20**:253-260. DOI: 10.1016/j.foodhyd.2005.02.017

[52] Hardenia A, Jayronia S, Jain S. Emulgel: An emergent tool in topical drug delivery. International Journal of Pharmaceutical Sciences and Research. 2014;**5**:1653-1660. DOI: 10.13040/IJPSR.0975-8232.5(5).1653-60

[53] Sengupta P, Chatterjee B. Potential and future scope of nanoemulgel formulation for topical delivery of lipophilic drugs. International Journal of Pharmaceutics. 2017;**526**:353-365. DOI: 10.1016/j.ijpharm.2017.04.068

[54] Mazumder B, Ray S, Kaurav S, Ghosh S, Dasgupta S. *In vitro* & *in vivo* studies on lornoxicam loaded nanoemulsion gels for topical application. Current Drug Delivery. 2014;**11**:132-138. DOI: 10.2174/ 15672018113106660063

[55] Vandana.2014.pdf, (n.d.)

[56] Mulia K, Ramadhan RMA, Krisanti EA. Formulation and characterization of nanoemulgel mangosteen extract in virgin coconut oil for topical formulation. MATEC Web of Conferences. 2018;**156**:01013. DOI: 10.1051/matecconf/201815601013

[57] Tarawneh O, Sunoqrot S, Hamed R, Basil M, AlBaraghthi T. Nanoemulsion-based gel formulation of diclofenac diethylamine: Design, optimization, rheological behavior and *in vitro* diffusion studies. Pharmaceutical Development and Technology. 2016;**21**:980-989. DOI: 10.3109/ 10837450.2015.1086372

[58] Srivastava M, Kohli K, Ali M. Formulation development of novel *in situ* nanoemulgel (NEG) of ketoprofen for the treatment of periodontitis. Drug Delivery. 2016;**23**:154-166. DOI: 10.3109/ 10717544.2014.907842

[59] Aithal GC, Nayak UY, Mehta C, Narayan R, Gopalkrishna P, Pandiyan S, et al. Localized in situ nanoemulgel drug delivery system of quercetin for periodontitis: Development and computational simulations. Molecules. 2018;**23**:1363. DOI: 10.3390/ molecules23061363

[60] Pathak MK, Chhabra G, Pathak K. Design and development of a novel pH triggered nanoemulsified in-situ ophthalmic gel of fluconazole: *Ex vivo* transcorneal permeation, corneal toxicity and irritation testing. Drug Development and Industrial Pharmacy. 2013;**39**:780-790. DOI: 10.3109/03639045.2012.707203

[61] Tayel SA, El-Nabarawi MA, Tadros MI, Abd-Elsalam WH. Promising ion-sensitive *in situ* ocular nanoemulsion gels of terbinafine hydrochloride: Design, *in vitro* characterization and *in vivo* estimation of the ocular irritation and drug pharmacokinetics in the aqueous humor of rabbits. International Journal of Pharmaceutics. 2013;**443**:293-305. DOI: 10.1016/j.ijpharm.2012.12.049

[62] Kaur G, Narang JK. Topical nanoemulgel: A novel pathway for investigating alopecia. Journal of Nanomedicine & Nanotechnology. 2018;**08**:6-10. DOI: 10.4172/2157-7439. 1000472

[63] Hosny KM, Banjar ZM. The formulation of a nasal nanoemulsion zaleplon *in situ* gel for the treatment of insomnia. Expert Opinion on Drug Delivery. 2013;**10**:1033-1041. DOI: 10.1517/17425247.2013.812069

[64] Setya S, Razdan BK, Talegaonkar S, Tariq M, Madaan T. Appraisal of transdermal water-in-oil nanoemulgel of selegiline HCl for the effective management of Parkinson's disease: Pharmacodynamic, pharmacokinetic, and biochemical investigations. AAPS PharmSciTech. 2017;**19**:573-589. DOI: 10.1208/ s12249-017-0868-0

[65] Wang Z, Mu HJ, Zhang XM, Ma PK, Lian SN, Zhang FP, et al. Lower irritation microemulsion-based rotigotine gel: Formulation optimization and *in vitro* and *in vivo* studies. International Journal of Nanomedicine. 2015;**10**:633-644. DOI: 10.2147/IJN.S74079

[66] Wei X, Senanayake TH, Bohling A, Vinogradov SV. Targeted nanogel conjugate for improved stability

and cellular permeability of curcumin: Synthesis, pharmacokinetics, and tumor growth inhibition. Molecular Pharmaceutics. 2014;**11**(9):3112-3122

[67] Aman RM, Hashim IIA, Meshali MM. Novel clove essential oil nanoemulgel tailored by Taguchi's model and scaffold-based nanofibers: Phytopharmaceuticals with promising potential as cyclooxygenase-2 inhibitors in external inflammation. International Journal of Nanomedicine. 2020;**15**:2171

[68] Tungadi R, Susanty W, Wicita P, Pido E. Transdermal delivery of snakehead fish (Ophiocephalus striatus) nanoemulgel containing hydrophobic powder for burn wound. Pharmaceutical Sciences. 2018;**24**(4):313-323

[69] Singka GSL, Samah NA, Zulfakar MH, Yurdasiper A, Heard CM. Enhanced topical delivery and anti-inflammatory activity of methotrexate from an activated nanogel. European Journal of Pharmaceutics and Biopharmaceutics. 2010;**76**(2): 275-281

[70] Elmataeeshy ME, Sokar MS, Bahey-El-Din M, Shaker DS. Enhanced transdermal permeability of terbinafine through novel nanoemulgel formulation; development, in vitro and in vivo characterization. Future Journal of Pharmaceutical Sciences. 2018;**4**(1):18-28

[71] Qian Q, Shi L, Gao X, Ma Y, Yang J, Zhang Z, et al. A paclitaxel-based mucoadhesive nanogel with multivalent interactions for cervical cancer therapy. Small. 2019;**15**(47):1903208

[72] Javed H, Shah SNH, Iqbal FM. Formulation development and evaluation of diphenhydramine nasal nano-emulgel. AAPS PharmSciTech. 2018;**19**(4):1730-1743

[73] Zakir F, Ahmad A, Mirza MA, Kohli K, Ahmed FJ. Exploration of a transdermal nanoemulgel as an alternative therapy for postmenopausal osteoporosis. Journal of Drug Delivery Science and Technology. 2021;**65**:102745

[74] Ma Q, Zhang J, Lu B, Lin H, Sarkar R, Wu T, et al. Nanoemulgel for improved topical delivery of desonide: Formulation design and characterization. AAPS PharmSciTech. 2021;**22**(5):1-4

[75] Mahtab A, Anwar M, Mallick N, Naz Z, Jain GK, Ahmad FJ. Transungual delivery of ketoconazole nanoemulgel for the effective management of onychomycosis. AAPS PharmSciTech. 2016;**17**(6):1477-1490

[76] Chin LY, Tan JYP, Choudhury H, Pandey M, Sisinthy SP, Gorain B. Development and optimization of chitosan coated nanoemulgel of telmisartan for intranasal delivery: A comparative study. Journal of Drug Delivery Science and Technology. 2021;**62**:102341

[77] Abioye AO, Issah S, Kola-Mustapha AT. Ex vivo skin permeation and retention studies on chitosan–ibuprofen–gellan ternary nanogel prepared by in situ ionic gelation technique—A tool for controlled transdermal delivery of ibuprofen. International Journal of Pharmaceutics. 2015;**490**(1-2):112-130

[78] Dhawan B, Aggarwal G, Harikumar SL. Enhanced transdermal permeability of piroxicam through novel nanoemulgel formulation. International Journal of Pharmaceutical Investigation. 2014;**4**(2):65

Section 3

Occular Drug Delivery

Chapter 4

Ocular Drug Delivery System: Barrier for Drug Permeation, Method to Overcome Barrier

Prakriti Diwan, Rajendra Jangde, Sulekha Khunte, Harish Bhardwaj and Preeti K. Suresh

Abstract

The physiological and anatomical barriers are major obstacles in the field of ocular drug delivery systems. The barriers involve nasolacrimal drainage, blinking, cornea, sclera, and blood-aqueous barriers whereas dynamic barriers involve conjunctival blood flow, lymphatic clearance and tear drainage. These barriers are showing natural protective functions, as well as limiting drug entry into the eye. Nanocarriers have been found to be effective at overcoming the problems and associated with conventional ophthalmic dosage forms. In this chapter emphasizes overcome to barriers and discusses advanced novel techniques used in the field of ocular drug delivery systems including nano dispersion systems, nanomicelles, lipidic nanocarriers, polymeric nanoparticles, liposomes, noisome, and dendrimer, have been investigated for improved permeation and effective targeted drug delivery to various ophthalmic site.

Keywords: ocular drug delivery, inflammation, conjunctiva, microphages, aqueous humor

1. Introduction

The eyes are one of the most important and complex sensory organs; they serve as a gateway for collecting and transmitting extraneous images to the brain as signals via the optic nerve. They maintain a relationship between the body and our surroundings through this action. Various disorders, such as inflammations or bacterial and viral infections, affect the eye's behavior. Such kind of disorders affecting the anterior eye tissues can be smoothly treated with high doses of drugs. However, diseases affecting the posterior tissue of the eye are tough to teach and treat. Age-related disorders including macular decay, glaucoma, diabetic macular edema, and proliferative vitreoretinopathies are some of familiar posterior eye diseases that can lead to vision loss if left untreated.

The complex structures of the eyes provide a high level of drug/treatment resistance. A thorough understanding of ocular anatomy, physiology, and barriers is essential for providing effective treatment for diseases affecting both anterior and posterior ocular tissues. This assists with clarifying the difficulties related with drug conveyance to eye. In this part, we give a point by point depiction of visual life systems and physiology as well as the blockade those stances difficulties to sedate conveyance.

2. Structure of the eye

The eye can be partitioned into two divisions the front fragment and the back section in structure of eye (**Figure 1**). The front fragment stays alive of the cornea, conjunctiva, watery humor, iris, ciliary body, and translucent focal point. These elaborate roughly 33% of the front of the eye. The leftover part for example back section made out of the sclera, choroid, Bruch's layer, retinal shade epithelium (RPE), nonpartisan retina, and glassy humor. An exhaustive depiction of the life systems and physiology of the eye is introduced beneath.

2.1 Cornea

The cornea is delicate, straight, smooth, vascularized, generally deciduous, and the most meticulous tissue in the body. The curved and rounded design allows it to be inserted directly into the external environment. The cornea develops in the white part of the eye called the sclera and the translucent tissue called the conjunctiva. The limitation of the cornea from which it connects to the sclera is known as the annulus. Limbus is strangely angiogenic and is thought to be a reservoir of pluri potent juvenile microorganisms. The surface of the cornea, which is not covered by the external environment, is invaded by the tear film, and its inner surface is mainly in contact with liquid called liquid humor. The thickness of the cornea often increases from the center to the periphery. These are seen in the twist of the cornea, which is huge in the center and has the smallest ring.

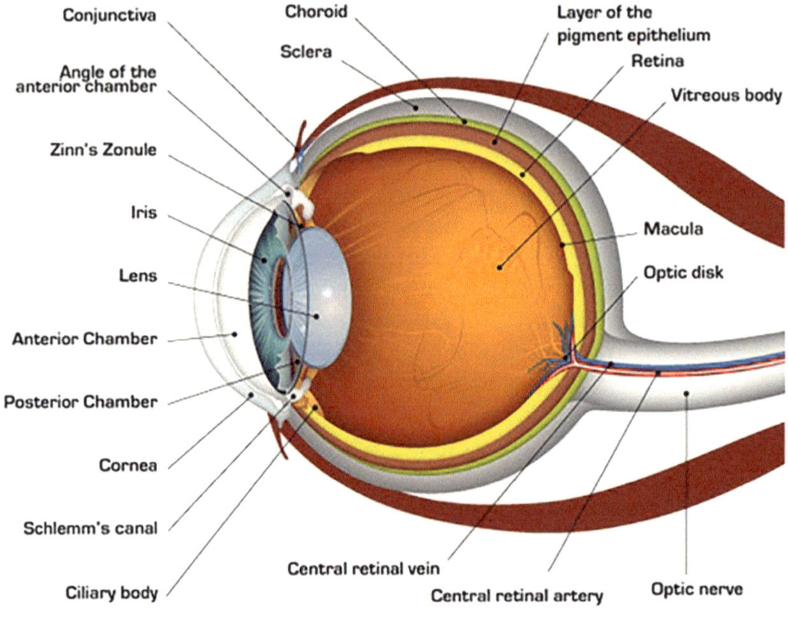

Figure 1.
Structure of human eye.

Corneal shape, surface perfection, straightforwardness, and refractive list manage the optical properties of the cornea. The corneal stroma is fixed with an almost homogeneous and methodical course of action of collagen fitters (distance across 25, 35 nm). Such a course of action is wanted to be answerable for forestalling and canceling dissipated light obstruction from the occurrence beam of light on collagen. The unequivocal plan and capacity of strands permit the light beams to ignore the cornea with next to no impedance. Corneal perfection is constrained by the corneal epithelium and tear film. Any redirection from the typical engineering of corneal collagen strands and nonappearance of tear movie inclusion causes dry eye and dissipating of episode light beams and prompts loss of corneal forms, straightforwardness, and perfection.

As mentioned above, the cornea is deeply attached to soft spots that are 300,400 times thicker than the skin [1]. Tactile nerves, long ciliary nerves, and well-thought-out involuntary nerve cords persuade the panniculus tissue. The ciliary nerve of the trigeminal nerve of the eye provides the tactile nerve to the membrane. The marginal nerve ring is formed by the longciliary nerve, which sheds its myelin sheath (at certain short distances) after entering the cornea, infiltrates the Bowman layer and then annihilate it with vane cells. These nerve cords further radiate anteriorly cross into the stroma, building the sub epithelial plexus [2]. Damage or loss of the corneal epithelium reveals external climate-sensitive areas. Causes extreme visual distress [3]. The typical cornea has no venous supply. Therefore, this tissue is treated as one of the internal tissues in the body along with ligaments and focal points. Internally, corneal epithelial cells and endothelial cells are metabolically dynamic and are effectively involved in injury healing. Both cell layers receive blood parts and various necessities from the veins of the internal and external carotid corridors that make up the conduit around the marginal cornea [4, 5]. Aqueous humor provides the cornea with the glucose it needs and a limited amount of oxygen. Most of the oxygenation of the cornea is evident in the opening to the air where the oxygen taken up by the lacrimal layer diffuses into the corneal epithelial cells. This openness of the saturated tear layer on the surface of the cornea is essential for oxygenation and maintenance of integrity and virtue. The histological section shows that the cornea is composed of six different layers, specifically the corneal epithelium, Bowman's layer, stromal, DNA layer, Descemet's membrane, and endothelium. The corneal epithelium is composed of 5–6 layers of discrete squamous epithelial cells that are not cornealized. The various epithelial layers of the cornea are composed of several layers of flat cells and wing cells and a single layer of basal cells. Various corneal epithelial cells are formed by rectangular parallelepiped basal cells with a tight cross-sectional structure that prevents tears from entering the intercellular space. After separation, these cells become delicately smooth as they migrate to the surface of the cornea. Electron microscopy shows that the outer layer of flat epithelial cells is sporadic and that rim-like disruption of the cell membrane is shown as microplica (**Figure 2**) [6]. This collapse expands the contact area. Microprica is covered with a very fine, tightly packed, charged sugar-coated layer that aids in scattering.

The fluid spreads evenly over the entire corneal surface at each strabismus. Flatepithelial cells are revived every 710 days by pluri potent microorganisms in the cornea llimbus [7]. More established cells are shed after their tight interface is destroyed by the tear film. The new cell layer controls tight junctions with the help of vane cells, which form lateral junctions between cells [8, 9]. Epithelial cells are connected to a 0.05 atm thick basement membrane consisting of columnar epithelium and are approximately 20 cm high. The presence of tight cells overlaps between the cell and the framework structure, and they are deeply impervious. Basal cells are the major corneal epithelial cells suitable for mitosis [10]. The Bowman's layer is a band of undefined fibrous material

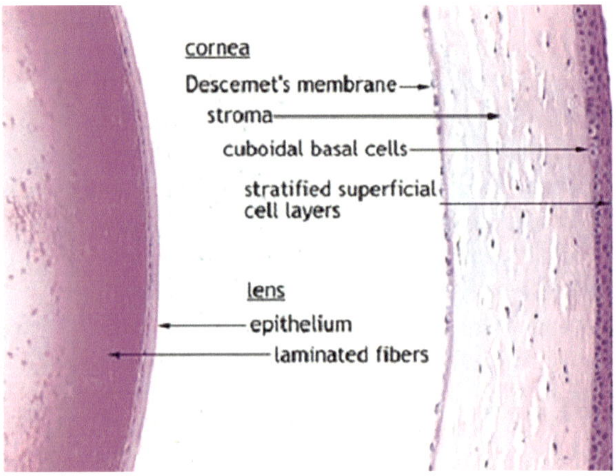

Figure 2.
Histology of corneal layer of the eye.

with a thickness of 81 Skm that simply resides beneath the base of corneal epithelial cells. This layer is non-regenerative, forming a boundary between the stromaof the cornea and epithelial cells and maintaining the shape of the cornea. It has been hypothesized that it is associated with re-epithelialization [11]. The Bowman layer is composed of short type I collagen fibrils embedded in the proteoglycan lattice. The stroma of the cornea intervenes between the Bowman layer and the Descemet's membrane and occupies 95% of the thickness of the cornea. The stroma contains corneal keratocytes, fibroblasts, brain tissue, and Schwann cells. Most of the interstitium is composed of collagen fibrils, mainly type I collagen [12]. These fibrils extend from one end of the annulus to the next and are calculated symmetrically at 90° in the anterior interstitium and symmetrically in the posterior interstitium. Collagen fibrils maintain the cornea with mechanical strength. The posterior interstitial fibrils are more tightly coordinated than the anterior, which clearly contributes to the mechanical and bipodal strength of the cornea [13]. The Dua's layer is a highly detailed, cell-free solid layer that resides on the Descemet's membrane [14]. Its physiological function in the cornea has not yet been investigated. The Descemet's membrane layer is 10 pm thick, the surface is undefined and huge. Upon invasion, this layer is alternative, homogeneous, cell-free and gradually transforms into Descemet's membrane [15, 16]. This layer is thrown into many creases that appear as stripes, because of awry enlarging of the back stroma, and underlying limitations name by the limbus.

The corneal endothelium is the most profound monolayers of cells, which is non-mitotic and in direct association with fluid humor, while endothelium control itself, stroma leftover in a deliquescent state to give corneal clearness [17]. This monolayer has characterized penetrability to particle transition, which is important to construct an osmotic angle. Endothelial cell numbers by and large downfall with age. During sickness, cells help in size (polymegathism) and show shape variety (polymorphism) to make up for the spaces made by declining cells.

2.2 Conjunctiva

Histologically, conjunctiva is primarily comprised shallow multifaceted epithelium and a fundamental stroma [18]. Conjunctival epithelial cells holds less close intercellular intersections with transepitlielial electric obstruction in the scope of 0.7S to −1.5 Kf2cm' [19, 20]. Conjunctiva moreover contains pores of 5.5 nm sweep [21].

Implanted inside the conjunctival epithelium are challis cells, mucous organs, organs of Manz and the sepulchers of Henle [22]. Challis cells are matched in electrolyte, liquid and bodily fluid discharge [23] to plan the tear film. Transportation of challis cells in various areas of conjunctiva persue a particular request: mediocre > predominant > nasal > fleeting conjunctiva [24]. The apical surface of conjunctiva shows out foldings called microvilli and microplicae [25]. During tear film part emission the conjunctival apical layer cells are breakdown alongside secretory granules and different parts into the tear film. Conjunctival apical out foldings might advance in expanding surface region, offer help or balance out and attach with tear film [25].

The conjunctiva is a thin, highly vascularized, opaque, mucous-draining tissue that covers the inner layers of the upper and lower eyelids [26]. It reflects off the eye as a faint, transparent tissue on the sclera and extends toward the annulus of the cornea. This tissue is very fast with efferent, afferent, tangible nerves, and also lymphoid tissue. The total surface area of the conjunctiva is many times the total surface area of the cornea [27, 28]. Due to its versatile nature, the conjunctiva promotes eye and eyelid movement. The lamina propria of tears combined with a small amount of aqueous humor protects the internal visual tissue from the external climate. Depending on the area, thickness, and angiogenesis, this tissue can be broadly divided into three types: eyelid, eyelid, and hamburger conjunctiva. The upper and lower eyelids are lined inside by a medium palpebral conjunctiva, with a small portion of the conjunctiva called the bulbous conjunctiva adjacent to the sclera. The bulbar conjunctiva is very light, standard on the cornea, and has open eyes with an air interface and is exposed to the outside climate (**Figure 3**). The eyelids and parts of the eyeball are connected by a small piece of tissue called the vestibular conjunctiva. The vestibular and volar conjunctiva are rich in veins and composed of heterogeneous tissue [26].

Conjunctival stroma is parleyed between the foremost epithelium and back sclera. This layer is equiped with blood and lymph vessels and innervated with sensitive spots. This is interlaced with mature lymphocytes, overwhelmingly with T cells comparative with B cells. Mucosa-connected lymphoid tissue assumes a urgent part in the resistant

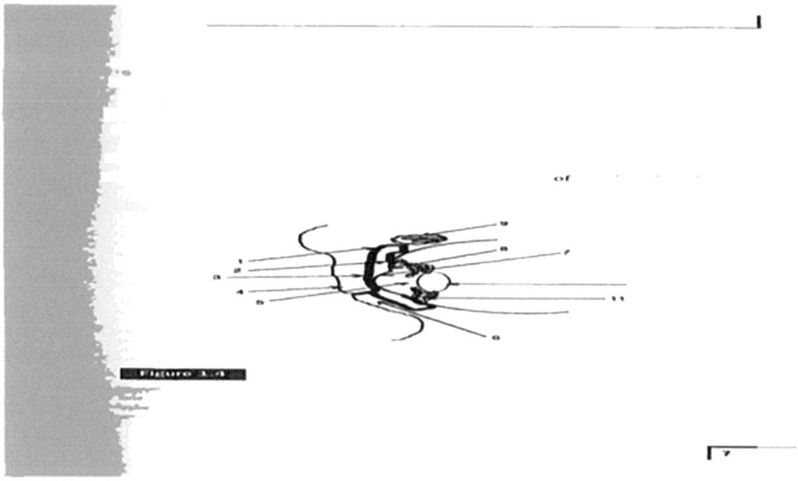

Figure 3.
Diagrammatic portrayal of front office of natural eye with shut eye covers showing three particular conjunctivas (striking layers). (1) Forniceal conjunctiva, (2) bulbar conjunctiva, (3) palpebral conjunctiva, (4) upper eye top, (5) watery humor, (6) lower eye lid, (7) cornea, (8) sclera and (9) lacrimal gland, (10) translucent focal point and (11) iris ciliary body.

reaction [29]. It is made out of lymphatic cells present underneath the epithelium, which achieve a safe reaction against antigens by emitting dissolvable antibodies. Lymphocytes are circled over particular vascular framework alluded high endothelial venules [30–32]. Electron micrograph of the tear film surface of the conjunctival epithelium. It shows (a) the mucous layer (m) and (b) the sugar coating (studs) present in the micropreca. (A) In this movie, we used various mucins, MUC1 (red), MUC4 (blue) and MUC1 (green). These protrude as solid bars to form the sugar coating from the microvilli of the epithelial cells. (B) The higher emphasis in the area (a) indicates fine fibers extending into the sugar coating (sharp stones), probably film-related mucin atoms. In the cytoplasm of microplica, actin fibers extend to the surface film, from which layered mucin emerges (giant bolts). (C) Small immunoelectron confinement of the immune agent H185 that senses carbohydrate epitopes on the layer-related mucin MUC16 [25].

2.3 Fluid humor

Watery humor is an optically clear, gently basic visual liquid that is developing from plasma by epithelial cells of ciliary body [33]. Three distinct cycles dissemination, ultra filtration and dynamic emission, commit to the compound organization and arrangement of fluid humor. It is anticipated that the whole watery humor is supplanted in roughly 100 min [34]. This liquid comprises somewhat less protein, egg whites and y-globulins, than plasma. Moreover, glucose, lactic corrosive, ascorbic corrosive and immunoglobulin G are similarly present [35, 36]. Fluid humor supplies supplements and an oxygen to the visual a vascular tissue, alluded as cornea and focal point. It clean up squanders items, macrophages, blood and other trash from the back of the cornea and front of the focal point. Additionally, it assumes a vital part in keeping up with the shape and interior afflictions of the eyeball over creation of intraocular pressure. The liquid humor that is assembled and drained into the posterior eye ignores the pupil in the anterior chamber. It is drained into the venous bloodstream through the trabecular meshwork and Schlemm's canal (**Figure 4**). Approximately 510% of the aqueous humor is used to secure the uveal scleral pathway [37, 38].

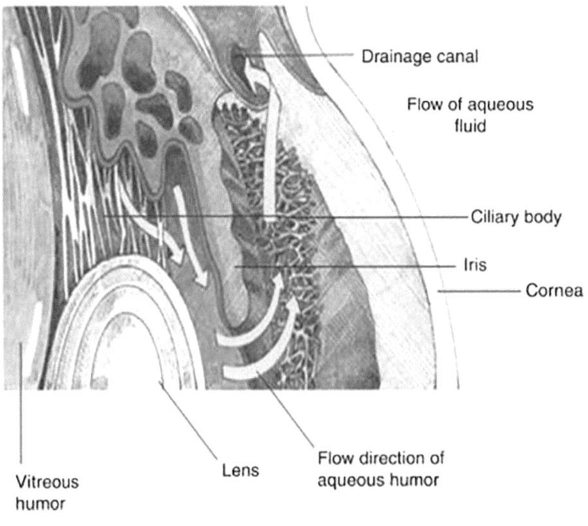

Figure 4.
Flow direction of aqueous humor from iris to canal of Schlemm or towards cornea.

2.4 Iris—ciliary body

The iris and the ciliary body are two distinct tissues with distinct physical and physiological properties. Their life systems and physiology are explained combined for simple mindfulness and close physical limits. The iris is placed at the back of the cornea and appears as a ciliary body spirit. The iris is made up of three layers: endothelium, stroma, and epithelium, according to histology. The iris creates a small roundabout opening or gap in the bleeding edge of the focus point, known as the student, which helps to control the amount of light that reaches the retina. Each ciliary body has a ciliary cycle, which conveys a fibrovascular core that is in continual contact with the ciliary body's stroma. Blood flow from the choroidal veins in the front to the back. The blood from the ciliary body of the eye is drained from the border of the vortex vein. The ciliary body is physically adjacent to the iris and is in charge of adjusting three vital capacities in the eye: it secretes watery humour, which runs before the focal point and is depleted out of the eye through tubules known as the trabecular meshwork and schlemm channel close to the intersection of cornea and iris (ii) this tissue also contains smooth muscles, which demonstrate through zonular filaments on the glasslike focal point to acclimate centigrade (iii) it can coordinate in emptying fluid humor out of the eye into the bordering trabecular meshwork by broadening smooth muscle strands and ligaments.

2.5 Focal point

The focal point is clear, internal, non-innervated and biconvex. It is situated behind the student and iris with the help of the ciliary body's zonular strands [39]. The foremost focal point is covered with fluid humor and the back with glassy humor. The focal point film (otherwise called the case) keeps up with latent trade of metabolic substrates and waste through straightforward dissemination [40] checked by their size and charge [41–44]. The focal point comprises of four explicit parts: the case, epithelium, cortex (fiber cell mass) and core. Additionally, it controls light passage into the eye and its refraction.

The case is an undisturbed, uncomplicated, versatile foundation layer that embodies the entire focus and provides the framework underlying the focus of the eye. Container thickness varies between species and within similar assemblies. For example, in mice, rodents, and rabbits, the container thickness is approximately 10 μm, 13 μm, and 14 μm, respectively. The thickness of the human front shell ranges from 25 to 30 μm compared to 14:00 on the back [45, 46]. A layer of casing protects the focus from direct contact with adjacent visual tissue and aqueous fluids. In addition, it acts as a sea of developmental factors, sequestering them [47–50] and forming a defensive barrier against microbial attack [51–53]. The arrival of developing factors from the container supports the improvement and isolation of focal cells. The instrument used to give the focal point its shape and surface curvature is fluffy. A tall, columnar monolayer of epithelium lies beneath the foremost focal vessel. The epithelium is not present behind the focal point in contact with the vitreous liquid. The cortex lies below the vessel and later in the epithelium of focus. It contains 68.6 of water [54]. The focal cortex is composed of newly assembled filaments that make up most of the focal point. The strands are tightly packed, the newly assembled filaments make up the nucleated organelles [2, 55, 56], and with age the strands shift towards the focal point (**Figure 5**) [46]. During this

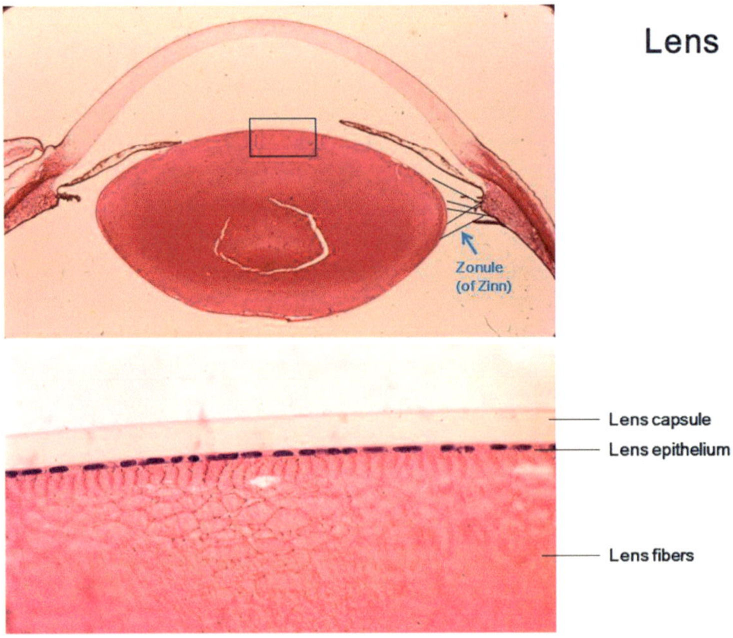

Figure 5.
Histology of lens.

development period, filaments lose organelles and nuclei, providing focus directness. The preparation of these filaments in adult focus involves four pointed stellar programs [57]. Entanglement between adjacent fiber cells can cause interlocks in deeper focal strands [57, 58]. Further migration to the focal cortex near the nucleus, the cells appear in the form of edgy hexagons. The locking system works together to even out the pressure during operation, perhaps preventing the fiber cells from slipping against each other.

The focal point core is exceptionally gotten by its area. It contains 63.4% water [54] and is started by testimony of old fiber cells that movement to the middle from the fringe. As the consequence of gathering of old cells in this zone, it turns out to be exceptionally thick and denser.

2.6 Sclera

The sclera, commonly referred to as the white of the eye, is a highly vascularized and flexible tissue beneath the conjunctiva and dilated cornea. The optic nerve exits the eye posteriorly through a scleral opening surrounded by a complex, grid-like, filamentous tissue network called the cribriform plate. The sclera (the top layer of the sclera) provides the expected nutrition to the sclera. The sclera occupies about 80% of the skin of the eye and the rest is composed of the inner cornea. Its physical area, the anterior sclera (near the annulus), thickens as it moves towards the equator, near and around the optic nerve, towards the back of the eye. It will decrease [59]. The sclera is composed of a sloppy tissue of filaments emanating from the dura mater of the focal sensory system. In this type of plan, all visible light frequencies are scattered and appear dazzlingly white in the shadows. At the interface between the sclera and the cornea, changes to true standard changes occur sporadically from nowhere, leading directly to such dark white scleral changes.

Similar collagen strands are available in the cornea yet are coordinated in a standard example that provisions straightforwardness to the tissue, hydrated sclera filaments stay obscure while corneal strands do not require water and become straightforward. The corneal endothelium serves to its straightforwardness by the droping out of water. Sclera, being the layer of the eyeball, is presenting to visit changes of outer alongside of intraocular pressure. Width of the sclera at tropical zone goes from 25 to 230 nm and at the fluid measurement of the sclera goes from 20 to 80 nm [60, 61].

2.7 Choroid

Choroid is put between fringe sclera and internal retinal epithelium. It is famously vascularized and innervated tissue fixing melanocytes alongside bodily fluid like extracellular liquid. It comprises of four particular parts: from external to internal suprachoroid, haller's layer, sattler's layer and Bruch's film. Suprachoroid is made by 6–10 layers, around 30 qm in which lay out the connection point between external sclera and internal [62]. The suprachoroid supported anteriorly with supraciliary and last posteriorly up to the optic nerve. This locale is exceptionally aroused with nerve strands and ganglion yet no vasculature. Meager lamellar filaments, in touch to one another, related the choroid and sclera. This procedure develops a small space between these tissues called the space on or around the choroid. This space is scarce as it moves backwards towards the macula.

The vascular layer below the supra choroid lamina is composed of three specific vascular layers, which are narrow and the distance within the lumen is continuously reduced. These blood vessels are surrounded by pigmented melanocytes and non-pigmented fibroblasts, reaching the maximum amount of choroid. Blood vessels, fibroblasts, and melanocytes appear in discreet amounts of choroidal stroma. The thickness of melanocytes increases from concentration to the periphery. Choroidal vessels are suggested by the luminal distance across the site as follows: Haller layer with larger outer blood vessels. Currently being tracked on a medium-sized vessel at Sattler's Layer. Well-traced choroid capillaries with narrowed blood vessels. Choroidal blood flow are also high in other visual tissues and the brain [63, 64]. The enlarged choroidal blood circulation provides an additional supply and diffusion of oxygen within the retina of the brain. Metabolic waste from the retina is carried away by changes in intraocular temperature caused by the visual cycle. This accelerated circulatory system also seems to predict sections when monitoring intraocular pressure [65–67]. Bruch's film is the last and deepest choroidal layer that covers the RPE [68]. Also known as the vitreous membrane. It is a thin, pentahedral, multifaceted, cell-free, layered structure initiated by the interaction of villous capillaries with RPE. Bruch's film grows from behind the eye, such as the optic nerve, to the oraserrata of the iris, with a continuous decrease in thickness from behind the eye to the edge. This film separates RPE and villous capillaries. Retinal cell associations include seven unique types of cells, including RPE cells. These are photoreceptor cells (poles and cones), squamous cells, amacrine cells, interstitial cells, bipolar cells, ganglion cells and glial cells (**Figure 6**).

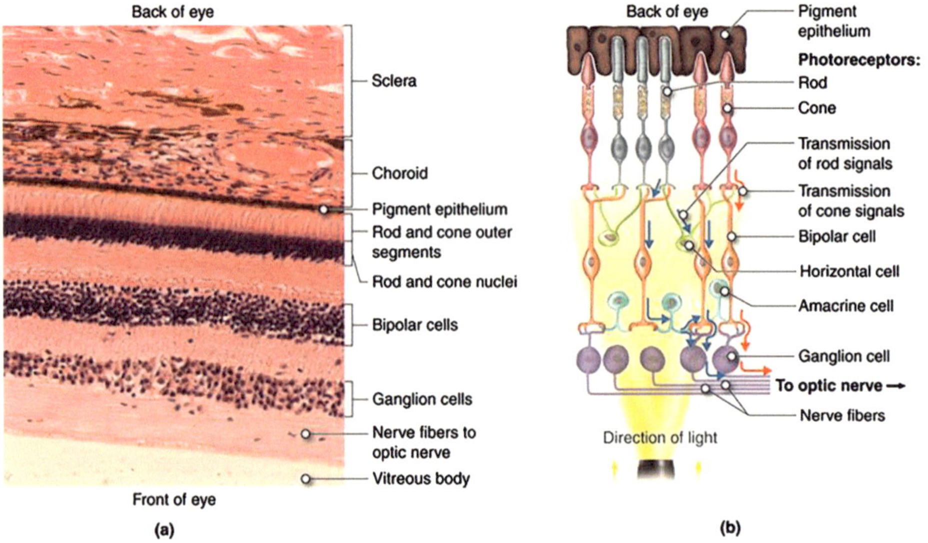

Figure 6.
Layers and histology of normal adult human retina.

2.8 Retinal pigment epithelium

Each individual eye contains approximately 3.5 million RPE cells [69], which attach to each other to form a narrow intersection (closed zone). The retina epithelium (RPE) contains non-dividing cells that form the monolayer that covers the retina of the cerebrum, but these cells can proliferate under masochistic conditions and are therefore isolated. I have not. It provides confirmation to the internal visual tissue and secretes large amounts of growth factors (vascular endothelial enhancer factor, ciliaryneurotrophin factor, and platelet engineering enhancer factor). This monolayer monitors visual resistance and protects against oxidative damage by releasing immune modulatory cytokines [70, 71]. RPE cells mediate several compounds such as superoxide dismutase, catalase, glutathione, and melanin clay. RPE supports the function of villous capillaries and photoreceptors and plays a fundamental role in patience. Therefore, its presence is important for the adjustment of visual boundaries [72]. Its capabilities include regulation of priotoceptors to external parts, retinoid processing, management of the visual cycle, and maintenance of sub retinal complex ecological variables [73–75].

2.9 Neural retina

Geologically, the retina is fashioned into macula, optic plate, fovea and fringe retina. The macula or are acentral is round 5 mm in thickness and positioned kind of three mm farfar from the optic circle. Macula accepts its call from the yellow carotenoid color ationxanthophylls, because the macula lutea. The focal factor of the macula serves a huge locale of visible sharpness [76] and is known as the fovea. The fovea has the maximum noteworthy thickness of confined and extended cone receptors to misrepresent mild location [77]. The focal factor of the fovea is vascular as much as 500 atm and the bloods deliver to this locale offers from chorio capillaries. Retinal fleeting veins encase the fovea. The outside layers of the fovea is thick and contain cores of photoreceptor cells. The relaxation fringe retina, bodily one layer of ganglionic cells, are to be had outside the fleeting retinal courses. Most outside retina receives its blood conveyances from the choroidal course, whilst standard retinal go with the drift satisfies inward retinal blood deliver [78, 79]. The inner arranging of the eyeball is made from mild-sensitive mind cells, alluded the mind retina, which talk tactile records to the cerebrum and interplay with the out of doors climate. These tactile nerves emerge from the focal sensory system [80, 81]. Brain retina is framed of round 7.7 million poles and five million cones (**Figure 7**) [82, 83]. The photoreceptor cells made from bars and cones. These cones basically ability to capture and extra de over the photons right into a nerve signal [84]. Retinal pole cells are accountable for keeping apart colorings in exquisite mild alien though cone cells has a tendency in keeping apart exceptionally contrasting shading in stupid mild. Biggest portions of cones are discovered with inside the fovea; whilst the bars are appropriated during the retina bar the focal fovea. The cones and bars are interconnected with among neurons named bipolar cells. Visual records is passing directly to ganglion cells through the a macrine cells, which cross approximately as an extension. Ganglionic cells talk records symptoms and symptoms to the focal sensory system, as an example mind. During power transmission Muller's telephonesassist in directing the community microenvironment for visible working.

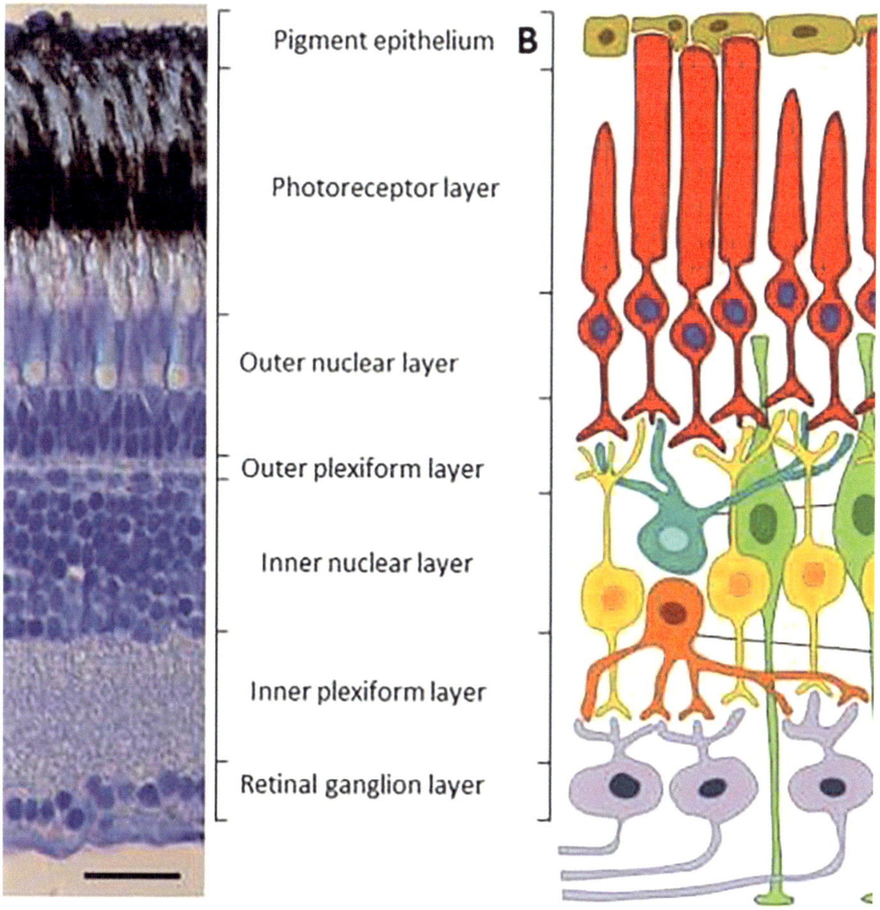

Figure 7.
Diagrammatic representations of rod and cone cells of neural retina.

2.10 Vitreous humor

The glassy humor is a straightforward, dismal, coagulated mass that consume the space in the eye between the focal point and the retina. It is encased by a layer of collagen named the glassy film (or hyaloid film or glassy cortex) isolating it from the remainder of the eye. It makes up four-fifths of the volume of the eyeball. The glassy humor is liquid like close by the middle, and gel-like close by the edges.

The glassy humor is in touch with the glassy film overlying the retina. Collagen fibrils associate with the glassy at the optic nerve circle and the oraserrata, (where the retina closes anteriorly), at the Wieger-band (the dorsal side of the focal point). The glassy likewise unequivocally connects to the focal point case, retinal vessels, and the macula, the region of the retina which gives better detail and focal vision [85].

Thickness of the liquid shrinkage with developing age. As this occurs, foremost watery humor might penetrate into the back glassy, bringing about a pulling impact at the association point of retina and glassy liquid. Moreover, this might source the arrival of cells into the liquid, which show up as floaters, and if a huge pulling impact is created it might pull off or withdraw the retina [86].

2.11 Hindrances to visual medication conveyance

Ophthalmic medications are accessible as arrangements, suspensions and balms, which are fundamentally directed topically. Elective courses of medication conveyance to the eye are oral, intravenous, intra vitreal, sub conjunctival and peri ocular infusions or inserts [87]. A challenge task in drug conveyance is to defeated visual boundaries and convey sedates definitively to the designated visual tissue. Drugs are meddling from arriving at designated visual tissues by static and dynamic natural visual boundaries. These obstructions can be ordered by their physical area and their practical properties. Generally, these obstructions can be named foremost and back section boundaries.

3. Front portion hindrances

There are two assortments of boundaries, for example static or dynamic boundaries. Static boundaries cover cornea, conjunctiva, iris-ciliary body, focal point, and blood watery boundary and efflux siphons propose on cell surface, for example, multidrug-safe proteins: penetrability glycoprotein. Conjunctival lymph, blood stream, inverse directional progression of fluid humor and tear creation together cover under the powerful boundaries. These obstructions are shown exhaustively underneath.

3.1 Cornea

The life systems and physiology of the cornea have been delineated before in this section. Cornea go about as a multifaceted mechanical obstruction to keep away from exogenous substances, including topically applied drugs, from infiltrating further into visual tissues. Expanding size influences the conjunctival penetrability. Bulbar and palpebral do not show a huge contrast [88]. Penetrability correlation that the conjunctiva is two times as porous as the sclera, while is roughly multiple times more penetrable than cornea. The epithelial pore size and thickness are two and multiple times more noteworthy in cornea and sclera individually. An anticipated complete paracellular space in conjunctiva is multiple times higher than that of cornea. External corneal layer, with 90% epithelium cells, convey this profoundly lipophilic. Mature corneal epithelial cells go about as a district for drug ingestion since they are firmly limited by cell bond, for example, Occludin, ZO1 and ZO2 [89]. These proteins tenaciously seal cells and establish a tight convergence for paracellular drug transport across the cornea.

Drug transport across films by a variety of devices, specifically (I) paracells, (II) transcellular, (iii) dynamic, (iv) carrier-mediated, and (v) receptor-mediated transport. Paracellular scattering of ionic (polar) particles is hampered by the narrow convergence of the cornea, but lipophilic preparations can be beneficially diffused through the transcellular portion across the lipophilic cornea. Bowman's shift does not have a significant impact on countering drugs with a wider distribution. Hydrophilic stroma is a rate-determining disorder of fat-soluble molecules, preventing more important visual media. In the case of a superbly lipophilic and almost hydrophilic combination, the epithelium and stroma act as a reservoir. Descemet'smembrane film is not involved in blocking drug intake on a regular basis. The corneal monolayer endothelium forms a cellular barrier between the stroma and the aqueous humor. This boundary mediates a flawed narrow intersection that promotes the free development of macromolecules between stroma and body fluids [90]. The distribution of drug intake through the cornea usually occurs in the aqueous humor. Subatomic size does not play an important role in transport through the corneal epithelium, but ionization of the mixture reduces transcellular dispersal. Therefore, particle physicochemical properties, ionization resistance, and visual medicine pH play important roles in maintaining and determining visual medicine porosity in the corneal epithelium 4. Vernal kerato conjunctivitis is a severely helpless conjunctivitis that impairs the dignity of the corneal epithelium and limits its prosperity. During this condition, eosinophils transport cytotoxic proteins such as myc-sponsored restricted protein (MBP1), eosinophil peroxidase, eosinophil-specific neurotoxin, and eosinophil-cationic proteins into the tears and the corneal epithelium. Reverse rotation of the epithelium [91–95].

Corneal ulcers are caused by the sensation of corneal fibroblasts by neutrophils. These fibroblasts are involved in the deterioration of nearby corneal collagen through various components such as disease putrefactive factors, interleukin 4, and interleukin 13 [96–98]. Therefore, the cornea loses an undeniable collagen strategy that can affect the corneal barrier properties against locally controlled drugs. Corneal fibroblasts are involved in the reverse rotation of collagen and can change parts of the basal layer to metastasize corneal ulcers. Tears from patients with vernal kerato conjunctivitis destroy type IV collagen and laminin, dominate part of the tornado protective layer, and accordingly lead to the development of corneal ulcers [99–102]. Conjunctiva Conjunctival tissue continues as a permeability limit to topically applied drugs. One of the limit properties can be connected with its transepithelial electric protection [103]. Various courses of prescription osmosis, for instance, paracellular, transcellular, dynamic and endocytic courses accept a key part in visual medicine transport through conjunctiva for topically applied drug things. The paracellular course of medicine immersion is noticeably bound in view of the presence of tight crossing points at the epithelial surface, which is the rate limiting development for drug maintenance [104]. The presence of secretory organs presented inside the conjunctiva could have a shock on drug osmosis [105, 106]. Tear creation is a careful response of the eye considering topically applied xenobiotics. A limit reduces the prescription concentration and bioavailability at the conjunctival apical surface. Physicochemical properties of the meds, for instance, hydrophilicity and subnuclear weight were found to accept a fundamental part in drug infiltration across conjunctiva. Test results explained that hydrophilic prescriptions with under 20 kDa nuclear burdens are vulnerable comparing higher subnuclear weight drug particles. By and large, conjunctiva has more conspicuous paracellular permeability than the cornea for proteins (insulin, subnuclear weight 5.8 kDa) and peptides (pamino clonidine subnuclear weight 245.1 Da) through its greater surface locale and defective vasculature [107, 108]. On the other hand, lipophilic prescription ingestion through the transcellular course has unequivocally higher responsibility relative with hydrophilic meds. As the conjunctiva has esterase activity [109], it could go probably as another impediment for drug transport. During the wiped out conditions the conjunctiva could expand and cultivate fibrosis as consequence of high proportions of collagen creation.

3.2 Blood liquid limit

Endothelial cells of iris/ciliary veins and the non-pigmented ciliary epithelium together arrangement the blood liquid limit (BAB) in the front piece of the eye. This prevention shapes tight convergences at the cell level and stays aware of the exchanging of solutes between the preeminent and back visual region. Thus, it hinders some vague medication entrance into more profound visual tissues by functioning as a boundary. Cell tight intersections blocks vague medication passage into internal visual tissues and proceed as an obstruction. BAB assists with managing visual straightforwardness and keeps up with synthetic substances structure [110, 111]. An ideal BAB conveys deficient obstruction usefulness; for instance, 40 kDa horseradish peroxidase arrives at watery humor through fenestrated ciliary vessels, which are associated with controlling penetration of plasma proteins, into the fluid humor. The vast majority of the medications arriving at watery humor are clear out into the fundamental course by means of the iris blood vessels. In this way, drugs in fluid humor are consumed by the iris colors and crash into the iris blood dissemination [112, 113]. Then again, little lipophilic medication atoms that withdraw tight intersections and cross BAB can be disposed of more quickly than the bigger hydrophilic particles. Accordingly, drug infiltration to more profound visual tissues is halted.

3.3 Efflux pump

Multidrug obstruction in cells might be to some degree created because of cell layer joined with efflux carrier proteins. These efflux siphons live from the adenosine triphosphate-restricting tape (ABC) superfamily and are effectively taken an interest in effluxing exogenous xenobiotics and cater insurance to the cell. Penetrability glycoprotein (P-gp) and multidrug obstruction protein (MRP) are two efflux proteins that are key members in drug efflux at the cell level, initiated a decreased intracellular medication fixation.

4. Front section dynamic boundaries

4.1 Tear seepage

Ophthalmic medication items are fundamentally managed by skin course into the visual circular drive. A huge segment (around 90%) of regulated drug is lost as the aftereffect of a precorneal obstruction—attack nasolacrimal conduits. Likewise, different variables that required into diminish drug focuses in the parkway incorporate tear weakening, drug restricting to tear proteins and sped up freedom.

Ordinarily, the advertised droppers are acclimated to convey a volume of effective drop from 20 to 50 μL. From the applied portion, the precorneal pocket contains just 7–10 μL by supplanting tear, which is as of now present in the precorneal pocket [114]. Such overabundance managed portion might be lost by means of spillage from the precorneal pocket or waste through the nasolacrimal pipe [115]. Precorneal tear waste washes the topically imparted drops/arrangements in the initial 15–30 s, causing a genuine decrease in drug contact time and finely lessening visual bioavailability <5 [116–118].

4.2 Conjunctival lymph and blood stream

The conjunctiva is immensely vascularized and equipped with lymph vessels. Topically applied drugs into the precorneal pocket may be essentially clear out into the fundamental and lymph dispersal while crossing the conjunctiva [119], achieving lower drug invasion to more significant visual tissue. Conjunctival blood and lymph stunningly limit the vehicle of sodium fluorescein from showing up at the inside retinal tissues [120, 121], exhibiting the effective work in drug end.

4.3 Watery humor

Watery humor produced by the ciliary body overflowing towards the cornea, the alternate way to the medicine entrance applied topically. Topically sedates, what separate across the front corneal epithelial may be also described by liquid humor stream. Meds may be exhausted out through trabecular meshwork into the channel of Schlemm. Greatest hydrophilic meds are seen as discard by watery humor using sub therapeutic levels in the inside visual tissues [122].

BAB activity can be abandoned due to immunological visual deterioration and can prevent reasonable vulnerabilities of experts on various subjects. Intravitreal monitored fluorescein-tested serum protein (FRSA) enters the main chamber after 5 min in the eye, but not in the control/abiotic eye [121]. It is worth noting that the basic fluorescein sodium particles actually pass through the BAB, but not the FRSA. The FRSA scattered in the first room seeks a two-step plan until it appears in the previous room in 23 h, generally with exorbitant obsession (Cmax). After that, the fluorescence continued to decrease. These preliminary results indicate that the student lost the boundaries of the BAB obstacle and lost dosing to the main chamber. In another audit, Kongetal. It has been shown that basic point-edge glaucoma damages the BAB and mediates irritation in the anterior part of the eye. Inconsistent reports between patients with severe terminal glaucoma (PACG) and patients with refractory PACG assume that patients with exceptional PACG have higher BAB damage than patients with consistent PACG [123]. It has been speculated that a significant increase in intra orbital load may be the causative variable for distinguishing BAB in the eye of PACG patients.

5. Posterior segment staticbarriers

5.1 Sclera

The sclera is one of the peripheral layers of the eye that cater security and forestalls the passage of exogenous substances to the back visual tissues. Porousness across sclera predominantly relies upon specific standards of the saturating particle, like atomic range, physicochemical properties and surface charge. Drug porousness across sclera steadily diminishes with expanding lipophilicity and sub-atomic span. Thus, particles with higher lipophilicity and bigger sub-atomic range might be kept from penetration through watery scleral pores. The contrary surface charge of the atom further restricts its pervasion across sclera. Drug atoms become caught in the pores of sclera causing low porousness presumably through connections with contrarily charged pores and proteoglycan network [3]. Scleral thickness varies as per their physical area. It is exceptionally wide posterior segment, close to the optic nerve because of its extensiveness; the back sclera has extremely low porousness for drug particles.

Bruch's shiftIn a sense, Bruch's film is concerned with directing the trading of dietary supplements, water, metabolic waste, oxygen, and biomolecules between the choroidal bloodstream and the retina [124]. Bruch's layer thickness increases with age, resulting in calcification, high cross-linking of collagen fibers, and turnover of glycosaminoglycans. The contrast in the thickness of this layer can also affect the permeability of the film from the sclera to the retinal tissue. Also, most medicines can enter the choroid before reaching Bruch's layer. In age-related conditions such as macular degeneration, extracellular edema and accumulation of edema result in oxidative pressure and inflammation of the Bruch layer. As extracellular flots and jets grow, the transport of supplements and drug atoms decreases. This may contribute to an increase in the metabolic pressure of the option [6, 123].

5.2 Blood retina obstruction

Blood retinal obstruction (BRB) consists of medial and lateral BRBs. The outer BRB is composed of tight junctions of RPE cells, while the inner BRB contains endothelial cells such as retinal hair. Tight junctions of the external BRB release retinal photoreceptors from the RPE [125, 126]. Two astrocytes and Muller cells provide the practical help expected at these narrow intersections. Together, these two cell types maintain the exchange of substances between the outer choroid and the inner retina. It supports astrocytes, catches up honestly, improves the occlusive properties of retinal endothelial blood vessels [127], and increases the safety of inward retinal cells so that they do not boil the flowing particles during retinal proliferation. The absence of windows on RPE and retinal endothelial cells is indistinguishable from blood brain obstruction and indicates potential drug distribution. RPE gives dissemination of tiny atoms like CO_2, O_2 and lipophilic particles to inward retinal tissues from the choroid. In this way, the boat of atoms might be intervened by receptor or energy/ATP-subordinate liquid stage pinocytosis. Thus, drug entrance is profoundly controlled because of the presence of tight intersections. Likewise, RPE go about as a siphon by getting dried out the sub retinal space. This includes keeping up with the ordinary neuro retinal pairing with RPE [128]. The siphon working is vital in light of the fact that there is no solid bond between the portions of outer brain retina and RPE. The inter photoreceptor framework, a gel-like thick arrangement happens between retinal cells, cause exceptionally powerless bonds. During the ischemic circumstances, retinal cement powers decline inside the space of minutes [129].

5.3 Efflux siphons

Transmembrane efflux siphons, for example, P-gp or MRP revealed on apical and basal sides of human RPE have been accounted for [130]. Articulation of P-gp on rodent retinal endothelial cells has additionally announced. Additionally, the presence of P-gp, MRP4 and bosom disease opposition.

protein in retinal vasculature of post pregnancy mouse was accounted for. The outflow of P-gp in retinal astrocytes was additionally been accounted for [131]. As of late, unique articulation levels of MRP1, MRP4 and MRP5 efflux proteins in human RPE cells have additionally been accounted for [63]. At cell level, these efflux siphons are energetically associated with diminishing the intracellular medication focuses and play out a significant obstruction to tranquilize conveyance.

5.4 Choroidal blood and lymph circulation

Choroid is an exceptionally vascularized tissue and outfitted with lymph vessels. This tissue has biggest blood vasculature (–80%) of the all out visual blood supply co-connected with iris-ciliary body and retina [7]. Lipophilic medication atoms are effectively depleted into the choroidal and fundamental dissemination, then, at that point, section into the inward visual tissues. This limited medication might prompt sub remedial medication fixation in retinal tissues. This limited medications entry might prompt sub helpful medication focus in retinal tissues. Studies with hydrophilic medications, for example, sodium fluorescein communicated extremely low end through choroid [8].

6. Ocular drug delivery systems

Visual medication conveyance framework there are principle issue of fast and exhaustive end of regular eye drops from the eye [9]. This issue brings about loss of enormous measure of medication. Just hardly any measure of medication enters the corneal layer and enter to inward tissue of eye [10, 11]. The primary explanation of medication misfortune incorporates lachrymal waste and medication weakening by tears [13]. This super smoothness diminishes the visual bioavailability and cause undesirable harmful and incidental effect. Yet, late biomaterials and nanotechnology headways have started a significant development in investigation into biodegradable microparticles and nanoparticles, hydrogel, and visual inserts, all of which can contain visual pharmacologic specialists, considering further developed prescription conveyance. Besides, supported discharge drug treatments might diminish the in general financial effect of visual sicknesses by lessening the aftereffects related with current clinical therapies [14]. Visual medication conveyance is progressing dangerously fast, on account of consistently advancing ways to deal with designated conveyance (**Table 1**).

6.1 Nanoparticles and microparticles

Nanoparticles and microparticles particulate polymeric medication conveyance frameworks comprise of miniature and nanoparticles. The prevalent size of microparticles for the ophthalmic organization in regards to 5–10 mm, over this size, a scratching sensation inside the eye might result after visual application. Microspheres and nanoparticles recommend excited drug transporters for ophthalmic application. The medication restricting depends on the physicochemical properties of the nano-or miniature molecule polymer. There after best medication restricting to those particles, the medication retention inside the eye is worked on widely when contrasted with eye drops. Particulates like nanocapsules, nanoparticles, nanosuspensions and so forth are wont to work on the bioavailability of visually applied drugs [15].

Brand name	Dosage form	Uses
Acuvail	4.5 mg/ml ketorolac tromethamine arrangement (0.45%) in a solitary use vial	Cataract medical procedure
Alocril	2% is an unmistakable, yellow, sterile solution	Allergic conjunctivitis
Elestat	0.05% epinastineHCl ophthalmic solution	Allergic conjunctivitis
Ozurdex	0.7 mg dexamethasone intravitreal visual implant	Retinal vein impediment
Pred Forte	prednisolone acetic acid derivation ophthalmic suspension, USP	Bulbar conjunctiva
Trivaris	80 mg/ml triamicinoloneacetonide injectable suspension	Sympathetic ophthalmia
Zymar	0.3% gatifloxacin ophthalmic solution	Bacterial conjunctivitis
Zymaxid	0.5% gatifloxacin ophthalmic solution	Bacterial conjunctivitis

Table 1.
Showcased product of ocular drug delivery system.

6.2 Fake tear inserts

In 1981 Merck, Sharp and Dohme was fostered an instrument for supported discharge alluded to as counterfeit tear. Industrially Lacrisert is out there inside the market. It contains hydroxyl propyle cellulose without additives used in the treatment of dry eye [132].

6.3 Visual inserts

In conventional arrangement of medication conveyance like suspension, arrangement and balm have various drawbacks. Visual additions limit the matter happen in customary framework. These are strong measurement structure have high ability to hold required convergence of medication in to designated tissue. A few examples of visual supplements are Dexamethasone, Pilocarpine nitrate, Tropicamide and Timolol Maleate [17].

Benefits of visual additions

A few benefits of visual addition which might be summed up as follows:

- Decrease of complete assimilation (which happens uninhibitedly with eye drops by means of the nasolachrimal channel and nasal mucosa).
- Likelihood of delivering drugs at a sluggish, consistent rate.
- Upgrade of visual residence, so that lengthy medication action and a raised bioavailability regarding regular vehicles.
- Right dosing (talk to eye drops which will be amazingly ingrained by the patient and are somewhat disappeared after organization, each addition are frequently made to contain a precise portion which is completely stayed at the organization site).
- Further developed time span with worship to fluid arrangements.
- Better persistent consistence, coming about because of compressed recurrence of organization and a lesser frequency of visual and foundational secondary effects.
- Plausibility of consolidating different novel substance/innovative methodologies.

6.4 Liposome

Liposomes are spherical phospholipids vesicles made up of one or more concentric bilayers arranged in a ring. They are non-toxic and biodegradable in nature, owing to the fact that they are made up of lipids that are similar to those found in biological membranes. Liposomes have the ability to entrap both hydrophilic and hydrophobic compounds in the aqueous compartments or the lipid layer due to their amphiphilic nature. Liposomes have a positive, negative, or neutral surface charge depending on their composition. Surface charge is one of the most important factors in liposome stability because it reduces the rate of aggregation and fusion during storage. The fact that the corneal epithelium is thinly coated with negatively charged mucin may explain why positively charged liposomes appear to be more important. Negatively charged liposomes are more effective than positively charged liposomes because of lowering of IOP over a longer period of time. The different structures and shape of liposome are classified;1. Multilamella vesicle (MLV): 520 lipid bilayer and very 5000 nm measurements 2. Oligolamera vesicle (OLV): 25 lipid bilayer and 1,001,000 nm measurements 3. Polyvascular vesicle (MVV): Very 1000 nm in diameter. 4. Single-layer vesicle (ULV): Single-layer of lipid Thesecan also be further categorized based on size potential 1. An SUV (more discreet single-layer vesicle) sized at 2040 nm. 2. MUV (medium-sized single-layer vesicle) with a size of 4080 nm. 3. 1,001,000 nm size LUV (larger single layer vesicle) 4. GUV (giant single-layer vesicle) with a size exceeding 1000 nm.

6.5 Collagen shield

Collagens have amazing biocompatibility and security in view of its natural attributes and for the most part used in clinical application since biodegradability and feeble antigenecity. Collagen safeguard was first ready from procine sclera tissues since they bear a collagens equal arrangement thereto of natural eye. The safeguards are hydrated before the inclusion into the eye commonly the medication is stacked into the medication answer for a time of at some point before application.

Collagen safeguard regularly produce a few uneasiness and obscured vision and are not fit every understanding. For improvement of this issue, Kaufman found a substitution idea of medication conveyance by combination of collagen safeguard particles and gets in-tuned with focal points named collasomes. Collasomes could be ingrained under the eyelid and limit the obscured vision issue [26].

6.6 Mucosal adhesive dose structure

In fact, mucosal adherent dose structures for visual delivery present many difficulties [24]. This approach relies on vehicles containing polymers that can bind to conjunctival mucin via non-covalent bonds. Mucoadhesive polymers are conventional polymeric hydrophilic colloids and contain several hydrophilic, practical compounds that can establish electrostatic bonds, similar to carboxyls, hydroxyls, amides, and sulfates. The bioadhesive metric structure showed higher drug bioavailability than the traditional dose structure. The effect of polyacrylicacid as a bioadhesive polymer on the visual bioavailability of timolol was evaluated. It has also been used to improve the visual bioavailability of progesterone [133].

6.7 Microemulsion

Microemulsions have local properties and a clear design. They are finished by automatic emulsification and disinfected directly. These assemblies have high drug dissolving capacity and excellent robustness. Due to these properties, it has excellent bioavailability. The mechanism of action of the drug is assimilation. Microemulsions contain nanospheres inside that hold the drug substance on the outer surface of the cornea and reduce drug waste [134].

6.8 Solution and suspension

These are liquid assemblies containing the active ingredients used in visual drug delivery. The drug substance must remain on the surface of the eye or in the internal area of the eye after passing through the cornea or conjunctiva. These arrangements even have some inconveniences such as unfortunate bioavailability and potency. Issues related to layout planning safety, bioavailability, and visual maintenance seasons are addressed through the work of a wide range of analysts by increasing thickness, using additives, and changing the pH of these definitions [28, 135].

6.9 Sol to gel systems

In 1980s a substitution idea delivering a gel set up was suggested by specialists. This thought of medication conveyance to eye is generally utilized in light of the fact that it expands the consistency and diminished the seepage of medication from cornea. Along these lines the bioavailability of medication naturally expanded. The in-situ gelling frameworks are regularly impacted by temperature, pH or particle enactment. In trial examination of bunny eye examiner found the in-situ gelling framework gives better and delay of medication contrast with the conventional eye drops [18].

7. Conclusion

The broad add visual medication conveyance during the sooner time frame. It's been plan, to expand the span of topically applied drugs inside the corneal and conjunctiva area. A few new methodologies like nanoparticles, liposome, contact focal points, visual supplements, collagen safeguard, set up initiated gel arrangement, non corneal course of visual medication dissemination, and nanoparticles-based polymeric arrangements and gels are being created by the drug science. An exhaustive depiction of the eye life structures and physiology, alongside its obstruction properties are given in this part. Perusers will be educated with various visual tissues, their physical areas, work and their static and dynamic hindrance nature. The natural eyes are fundamental and biggest delicate and profoundly watched organs in the body. These are extremely confounded organs and which are immediate contact with the outside conditions, this organ is truly helpless against injury and subsequently impermeable to exogenous synthetic compounds. In addition, over the top tear creation in view of reaction to outer upgrades or remedial specialists and furthermore expanded flickering rate due to adding to shield. These security capacities normally created and go about as an obstruction to remotely applied drugs, particularly when these are designated to tissues at the rear of the eye. Articulation of medication efflux siphons at a cell level squares drug section into the sick cell and afterward presents serious difficulties to visual medication conveyance. The physicochemical properties of the medication and conveyance framework can be arched relying upon the designated eye tissue. For the back eye conveyance, different courses of medication organization, for example, periocular infusions/inserts, are successfully utilized to defeat visual static and dynamic boundaries. Accordingly, information on the different visual tissues alongside the dynamic drug and physicochemical boundary properties is vital. The data gave in this part might facilitate the improvement of an ideal definition for designated conveyance.

Author details

Prakriti Diwan, Rajendra Jangde*, Sulekha Khunte, Harish Bhardwaj and Preeti K. Suresh
University Institute of Pharmacy, Pt. Ravishankar Shukla University, Raipur, C.G., India

*Address all correspondence to: rjangdepy@gmail.com

References

[1] Patton TF, Robinson JR. Quantitative precorneal disposition of topically applied pilocarpine nitrate in rabbit eyes. Journal of Pharmaceutical Sciences. 1976;**65**(9):1295-1301

[2] Wood RW, Li VH, Kreuter J, Robinson JR. Ocular disposition of poly-hexyl-2-cyano [3-14C] acrylate nanoparticles in the albino rabbit. International Journal of Pharmaceutics. 1985;**23**(2):175-183

[3] Lee VHL, Robinson JR. Mechanistic and quantitative evaluation of precornealpilocarpine disposition in albino rabbits. Journal of Pharmaceutical Sciences. 1979;**68**(6):673-684

[4] Joshi A, Ding S, Himmelstein KJ. Reversible gelatin composition and method of use. US Patent No. 5,252,318; October 12 1993

[5] Kumar S, Haglund BO, Himmelstein KJ. In situ-forming gels for ophthalmic drug delivery. Journal of Ocular Pharmacology and Therapeutics. 1994;**10**(1):47-56

[6] Keister JC, Cooper ER, Missel PJ, Lang JC, Hager DF. Limits on optimizing ocular drug delivery. Journal of Pharmaceutical Sciences. 1991;**80**(1):50-53

[7] Lee VL. Precorneal, corneal, and postcorneal factors. Drugs and the Pharmaceutical Sciences. 1993;**58**:59-81

[8] Tang NE, Zuure PL, Pardo RD, de Keizer RJ, Van Best JA. Reflex lacrimation in patients with glaucoma and healthy control subjects by fluorophotometry. Investigative Ophthalmology & Visual Science. 2000;**41**(3):709-714

[9] White WL, Glover AT, Buckner AB. Effect of blinking on tear elimination as evaluated by dacryoscintigraphy. Ophthalmology. 1991;**98**(3):367-369

[10] Stewart WC. Review timolol hemihydrate: A new formulation of Timolol for the treatment of glaucoma. Journal of Ocular Pharmacology and Therapeutics. 1996;**12**(2):225-237

[11] Ahmed I, Patton TF. Importance of the noncorneal absorption route in topical ophthalmic drug delivery. Investigative Ophthalmology & Visual Science. 1985;**26**(4):584-587

[12] Schoenwald RD, Deshpande GS, Rethwisch DG, Barfknecht CF. Penetration into the anterior chamber via the conjunctival/scleral pathway. Journal of Ocular Pharmacology and Therapeutics. 1997;**13**(1):41-59

[13] Mishima S, Gasset A, Klyce SD, Baum JL. Determination of tear volume and tear flow. Investigative Ophthalmology & Visual Science. 1966;**5**(3):264-276

[14] Chrai SS, Patton TF, Mehta A, Robinson JR. Lacrimal and instilled fluid dynamics in rabbit eyes. Journal of Pharmaceutical Sciences. 1973;**62**(7):1112-1121

[15] allergan.com

[16] Sikandar MK, Sharma PK, Visht S. Ocular drug delivery system: An overview. International Journal of Pharmaceutical Sciences and Research. 2011;**2**(5):1168

[17] LaMotte J, Grossman E, Hersch J. The efficacy of cellulosic ophthalmic inserts for treatment of dry eye. Journal of the American Optometric Association. 1985;**56**(4):298-302

[18] Rootman DS, Jantzen JA, Gonzalez JR, Fischer MJ, Beuerman R, Hill JM. Pharmacokinetics and safety of transcornealiontophoresis of tobramycin in the rabbit. Investigative Ophthalmology & Visual Science. 1988;**29**(9):1397-1401

[19] Nagarsenker MS, Londhe VY, Nadkarni GD. Preparation and evaluation of liposomal formulations of tropicamide for ocular delivery. International Journal of Pharmaceutics. 1999;**190**(1):63-71

[20] Mitra AK. Ophthalmic Drug Delivery Systems. 2003

[21] Hui HW, Robinson JR. Ocular delivery of progesterone using a bioadhesive polymer. International Journal of Pharmaceutics. 1985;**26**(3):203-213

[22] Vandamme TF. Microemulsions as ocular drug delivery systems: Recent developments and future challenges. Progress in Retinal and Eye Research. 2002;**21**(1):15-34

[23] Mueller WH, Deardorff DL. Ophthalmic vehicles: The effect of methylcellulose on the penetration of homatropinehydrobromide through the cornea. Journal of the American Pharmaceutical Association. 1956;**45**(5):334-341

[24] Krishna N, Brow F. Polyvinyl alcohol as an ophthalmic vehicle: Effect on regeneration of corneal epithelium. American Journal of Ophthalmology. 1964;**57**(1):99-106

[25] Middleton DL, Robinson JR. Design and evaluation of an ocular bioadhesive delivery system. STP Pharma Sciences. 1991;**1**(3):200-206

[26] Lerman S, Davis P, Jackson WB. Prolonged release hydrocortisone therapy. Canadian Journal of Ophthalmology. Journal CanadienD'ophtalmologie. 1973;**8**(1):114-118

[27] Karthikeyan D, Bhowmick M, Pandey VP, Nandhakumar J, Sengottuvelu S, Sonkar S, et al. The concept of ocular inserts as drug delivery systems: An overview. Asian Journal of Pharmaceutics (AJP). 2014;**2**(4)

[28] Vadnere M, Amidon G, Lindenbaum S, Haslam JL. Thermodynamic studies on the gel-sol transition of some pluronicpolyols. International Journal of Pharmaceutics. 1984;**22**(2-3):207-218

[29] Worakul N, Robinson JR. Ocular pharmacokinetics/pharmacodynamics. European Journal of Pharmaceutics and Biopharmaceutics. 1997;**44**(1):71-83

[30] McGhee PCN. An Overview of Topical Ophthalmic Drugs and the Therapeutics of Ocular Infection. CNJ Mc Ghee: Ocular Therapeutics. 2017

[31] Jitendra SP, Banik A, Dixit S. A new trend: Ocular drug delivery system. International. Journal of Pharmaceutical Sciences. 2011;**2**(3):720-744

[32] Patel A, Cholkar K, Agrahari V, Mitra AK. Ocular drug delivery systems: An overview. World Journal of Pharmacology. 2013;**2**(2):47

[33] Urtti A. Challenges and obstacles of ocular pharmacokinetics and drug delivery. Advanced Drug Delivery Reviews. 2006;**58**(11):1131-1135

[34] Galloway NR. Common eye diseases and their management. American Journal of Ophthalmology. **100**(2):360

[35] Ng JS. Ocular anatomy and physiology. Optometry & Vision Science. 2009;**86**(10):1208

[36] Gaudana R, Ananthula HK, Parenky A, Mitra AK. Ocular drug delivery. The AAPS Journal. 2010;**12**(3):348-360

[37] Khurana VK, Agrahari V. Recent advances in ocular drug delivery. Advanced Drug Delivery. 2014. (Chapter 19)

[38] Barar J, Asadi M, Mortazavi-Tabatabaei SA, Omidi Y. Ocular drug delivery; impact of in vitro cell culture models. Journal of Ophthalmic & Vision Research. 2009;**4**(4):238

[39] Achouri D, Alhanout K, Piccerelle P, Andrieu V. Recent advances in ocular drug delivery. Drug development and industrial pharmacy. 2013;**39**(11):1599-1617

[40] Barar J, Javadzadeh AR, Omidi Y. Ocular novel drug delivery: Impacts of membranes and barriers. Expert Opinion on Drug Delivery. 2008;**5**(5):567-581

[41] Ghate D, Edelhauser HF. Ocular drug delivery. Expert Opinion on Drug Delivery. 2006;**3**(2):275-287

[42] Ruponen M, Urtti A. Undefined role of mucus as a barrier in ocular drug delivery. European Journal of Pharmaceutics and Biopharmaceutics: Official Journal of Arbeitsgemeinschaft fur PharmazeutischeVerfahrenstechnik eV. 2015;**96**:442-446

[43] Gaudana R, Jwala J, Boddu SH, Mitra AK. Recent perspectives in ocular drug delivery. Pharmaceutical Research. 2009;**26**(5):1197-1216

[44] Anand BS, Dey S, Mitra AK. Current prodrug strategies via membrane transporters/receptors. Expert Opinion on Biological Therapy. 2002;**2**(6):607-620

[45] Kaur IP, Garg A, Singla AK, Aggarwal D. Vesicular systems in ocular drug delivery: An overview. International Journal of Pharmaceutics. 2004;**269**(1):1-14

[46] Du Toit LC, Pillay V, Choonara YE, Govender T, Carmichael T. Ocular drug delivery—A look towards nanobioadhesives. Expert Opinion on Drug Delivery. 2011;**8**(1):71-94

[47] Djebli N, Khier S, Griguer F, Coutant AL, Tavernier A, Fabre G. Ocular drug distribution after topical administration: Population pharmacokinetic model in rabbits. European Journal of Drug Metabolism and Pharmacokinetics. 2016

[48] Siegal. Glaucoma Medical Therapy: Principles and Management: Principles and Management. 2008

[49] Dua HS, Faraj LA, Said DG, Gray T, Lowe J. Human corneal anatomy redefined: A novel pre-Descemet's layer (Dua's layer). Ophthalmology. 2013;**20**(9):1778-1785

[50] Almeida H, Amaral MH, Lobao P, Lobo JM. In situ gelling systems: A strategy to improve the bioavailability of ophthalmic pharmaceutical formulations. Drug Discovery Today. 2014;**19**(4):400-412

[51] Salazar MM, Wainer I, Patil PN. Relevance of drug-melanin interactions to ocular pharmacology and toxicology. Journal of Ocular Pharmacology. 1994;**10**(1):217-239

[52] Barot M, Patel M, Kwatra D, Mitra AK. 7—Transporter–metabolism interplay in the eye. In: Ocular Transporters and Receptors. Woodhead Publishing; 2013. pp. 229-248

[53] Dhananjay P, Krishna RV, AswaniDutt V, Mitra AK. Biology of ocular transporters: Efflux and influx transporters in the eye. In: Ocular Transporters and Receptors. WoodheadPublishing; 2013. pp. 37-84

[54] Maurice D. Practical issues in intravitreal drug delivery. Journal of Ocular Pharmacology and Therapeutics:

The Official Journal of the Association for Ocular Pharmacology and Therapeutics. 2001;**17**(4):393-401

[55] Raghava S, Hammond M, Kompella UB. Periocular routes for retinal drug delivery. Expert Opinion on Drug Delivery. 2004;**1**(1):99-114

[56] OkadaAA,WakabayashiT,MorimuraY, Kawahara S, Kojima E, Asano Y. Trans-Tenon'sretrobulbar triamcinolone infusion for the treatment of uveitis. The British Journal of Ophthalmology. 2003;**87**(8):968-971

[57] Johnson KS, Chu DS. Evaluation of sub-Tenon triamcinolone acetonide injections in the treatment of scleritis. American Journal of Ophthalmology. 2010;**149**(1):77-81

[58] Chang DT, Herceg MC, Bilonick RA, Camejo L, Schuman JS, Noecker RJ. Intracameral dexamethasone reduces inflammation on the first postoperative day after cataract surgery in eyes with and without glaucoma, Clinicalophthalmology. 2009;**3**:345-355

[59] Mishima S. Clinical pharmacokinetics of the eye: Proctor lecture. Investigative Ophthalmology & Visual Science. 1981;**21**(4):504-541

[60] Le Bourlais C, Acar L, Zia H, Sado PA, Needham T, Leverge R. Ophthalmic drug delivery systems—Recent advances. Progress in Retinal and Eye Research. 1998;**17**(1):33-58

[61] Urtti A, Salminen. Minimizing systemic absorption of topically administered ophthalmic drugs. Survey of Ophthalmology. 1993;**37**(6):435-456

[62] Benedetti MS, Whomsley R, Poggesi I, Cawello W, Mathy FX, Delporte ML. Drug metabolism and pharmacokinetics. Drug Metabolism Reviews. 2009;**41**(3):344-390

[63] Tangri P, Khurana S. Basics of ocular drug delivery systems. International Journal of Research in Pharmaceutical and Biomedical Sciences. 2011;**2**(4):1541-1552

[64] Katragadda S, Gunda S, Hariharan S, Mitra AK. Ocular pharmacokinetics of acyclovir amino acid ester prodrugs in the anterior chamber: Evaluation of their utility in treating ocular HSV infections. International Journal of Pharmaceutics. 2008;**359**(1-2):15-24

[65] Levison ME, Levison JH. Pharmacokinetics and pharmacodynamics of antibacterial agents. Infectious Disease Clinics of North America. 2009;**23**(4):791-815

[66] Del Amo EM, Urtti A. Rabbit as an animal model for intravitreal pharmacokinetics: Clinical predictability and quality of the published data. Experimental Eye Research. 2015;**137**:111-124

[67] Bartlett JD, Jaanus SD. Clinical Ocular Pharmacology. St. Louis: Butterworth-Heinemann/Elsevier; 2008

[68] Novack GD, Robin AL. Ocular pharmacology. Journal of Clinical Pharmacology. 2016;**56**(5):517-527

[69] Vellonen KS, Soini EM, Amo EM, Urtti A. Prediction of ocular drug distribution from systemic blood circulation. Molecular Pharmaceutics. 2015

[70] Tojo K. Pharmacokinetic model for ocular drug delivery. Chemical & Pharmaceutical Bulletin. 2004;**52**(11):1290-1294

[71] Chiou GC. Systemic delivery of polypeptide drugs through ocular route. Journal of Ocular Pharmacology. 1994;**10**(1):93-99

[72] Makoid MC, Robinson JR. Pharmacokinetics of topically applied

pilocarpine in the albino rabbit eye. Journal of Pharmaceutical Sciences. 1979;**68**(4):435-443

[73] Fauser S, Kalbacher H, Alteheld N, Koizumi K, Krohne TU, Joussen AM. Pharmacokinetics and safety of intravitreally delivered etanercept. Graefe'sArchive for Clinical and Experimental Ophthalmology Albrecht von Graefes Archiv fur klinische undexperimentelleOphthalmologi. 2004;**242**(7):582-586

[74] Iyer MN, He F, Wensel TG, Mieler WF, Benz MS, Holz ER. Intravitreal clearance of moxifloxacin. Transactions of the American Ophthalmological Society. 2005;**103**:76-81. discussion 3

[75] BakriSJ,SnyderMR,ReidJM,PulidoJS, Ezzat MK, Singh RJ. Pharmacokinetics of intravitrealranibizumab (Lucentis). Ophthalmology. 2007;**114**(12):2179-2182

[76] Wu CY, Wu HM, Lee JD, Weng HH. Stroke risk factors and subtypes in different age groups: A hospital-based study. Neurology India. 2010;**58**(6):863-868

[77] Xu L, Lu T, Tuomi L, Jumbe N, Lu J, Eppler S. Pharmacokinetics of ranibizumab in patients with neovascular age-related macular degeneration: A population approach. Investigative Ophthalmology & Visual Science. 2013;**54**(3):1616-1624

[78] Gaudreault J, Fei D, Rusit J, Suboc P, Shiu V. Preclinical pharmacokinetics of Ranibizumab (rhuFabV2) after a single intravitreal administration. Investigative Ophthalmology & Visual Science. 2005;**46**(2):726-733

[79] Proksch JW, Lowe ER, Ward KW. Ocular pharmacokinetics of mapracorat, a novel, selective glucocorticoid receptor agonist, in rabbits and monkeys. Drug Metabolism and Disposition: The Biological Fate of Chemicals. 2011;**39**(7):1181-1187

[80] Le KN, Gibiansky L, Good J, Davancaze T, van Lookeren CM, Loyet KM. A mechanistic pharmacokinetic/pharmacodynamic model of factor D inhibition in cynomolgus monkeys by lampalizumab for the treatment of geographic atrophy. The Journal of Pharmacology and Experimental Therapeutics. 2015;**355**(2):288-296

[81] Drolet DW, Nelson J, Tucker CE, Zack PM, Nixon K, Bolin R. Pharmacokinetics and safety of an anti-vascular endothelial growth factor aptamer (NX1838) following injection into the vitreous humor of rhesus monkeys. Pharmaceutical Research. 2000;**17**(12):1503-1510

[82] Tucker CE, Chen LS, Judkins MB, Farmer JA, Gill SC, Drolet DW. Detection and plasma pharmacokinetics of an anti-vascular endothelial growth factor oligonucleotide-aptamer (NX1838) in rhesus monkeys. Journal of Chromatography B, Biomedical Sciences and Applications. 1999;**732**(1):203-212

[83] Ng EW, Shima DT, Calias P, Cunningham ET, Guyer DR, Adamis AP. Targeted anti-VEGF aptamer for ocular vascular diseas. Nature Reviews Drug Discovery. 2006;**5**(2):123-132

[84] Liu YC, Peng Y, Lwin NC, Wong TT, Venkatraman SS, Mehta JS. Optimization of subconjunctival biodegradable microfilms for sustained drug delivery to the anterior segment in a small animal model. Investigative Ophthalmology & Visual Science. 2013;**54**(4):2607-2615

[85] Di Tommaso C, Bourges JL, Valamanesh F, Trubitsyn G, Torriglia A,

Jeanny JC. Novel micelle carriers for cyclosporin A topical ocular delivery: In vivo cornea penetration, ocular distribution and efficacy studies. European Journal of Pharmaceutics and Biopharmaceutics: Official Journal of Arbeitsgemeinschaft fur PharmazeutischeVerfahrenstechnikeV. 2012;**81**(2):257-264

[86] Hendrix DV, Stuffle JL, Cox SK. Pharmacokinetics of topically applied ciprofloxacin in equine tears. Veterinary Ophthalmology. 2007;**10**(6):344-347

[87] Proksch JW, Granvil CP, Siou-MermetR,ComstockTL,PaternoMR, Ward KW. Ocular pharmacokinetics of besifloxacin following topical administration to rabbits, monkeys, and humans. Journal of Ocular Pharmacology and Therapeutics. The Official Journal of the Association for Ocular Pharmacology and Therapeutics. 2009;**25**(4):335-344

[88] Shen J, Durairaj C, Lin T, Liu Y, Burke J. Ocular pharmacokinetics of intravitreally administered brimonidine and dexamethasone in animal models with and without blood-retinal barrier breakdown. Investigative Ophthalmology & Visual Science. 2014;**55**(2):1056-1066

[89] Kymionis GD, Bouzoukis DI, Diakonis VF, Siganos C. Treatment of chronic dry eye: Focus on cyclosporine. Clinical Ophthalmology. 2008;**2**(4):829-836

[90] Mathews D, Mathews J, Jones NP. Low-dose cyclosporine treatment for sight-threatening uveitis: Efficacy, toxicity, and tolerance. Indian Journal of Ophthalmology. 2010;**58**(1):55-58

[91] Tang-Liu DD, Acheampong A. Ocular pharmacokinetics and safety of ciclosporin, a novel topical treatment for dry eye. Clinical Pharmacokinetics. 2005;**44**(3):247-261

[92] Bucolo C, Melilli B, Piazza C, Zurria M, Drago F. Ocular pharmacokinetics profile of different indomethacin topical formulations. Journal of Ocular Pharmacology and Therapeutics: The Official Journal of the Association for Ocular Pharmacology and Therapeutics. 2011;**27**(6):571-576

[93] Amar T, Caillaud T, Elena PP. Ocular pharmacokinetic study following single and multiple azithromycin administrations in pigmented rabbits. Current Eye Research. 2008;**33**(2):149-158

[94] Akpek EK, Vittitow J, Verhoeven RS, Brubaker K, Amar T, Powell KD. Ocular surface distribution and pharmacokinetics of a novel ophthalmic 1% azithromycin formulation. Journal of Ocular Pharmacology and Therapeutics: The Official Journal of the Association for Ocular Pharmacology and Therapeutics. 2009;**25**(5):433-439

[95] Johannesson G, Moya MD, Asgrimsdottir GM, Lund SH, Thorsteinsdottir M, Loftsson T. Kinetics of gamma-cyclodextrin nanoparticle suspension eye drops in tear fluid. ActaOphthalmologica. 2014;**92**(6):550-556

[96] Amon M, Busin M. Efficacy and safety for postoperative anti-inflammatory use. International Ophthalmology. 2012;**32**(5):507-517

[97] Schopf L, Enlow E, Popov A, Bourassa J, Chen H. Ocular pharmacokinetics of a novel LoteprednolEtabonate 0.4% ophthalmic formulation. Ophthalmology and Therapy. 2014

[98] Kapanigowda UG, Nagaraja SH, Ramaiah B, Boggarapu PR. Improved intraocular bioavailability of ganciclovir by mucoadhesive polymer based ocular

microspheres: Development and simulation process in Wistar rats. Daru: Journal of Faculty of Pharmacy, Tehran University of Medical Sciences. 2015;**23**(1):49

[99] Bakri SJ, Snyder MR, Reid JM, Pulido JS, Singh RJ. Pharmacokinetics of intravitrealbevacizumab (Avastin). Ophthalmology. 2007;**114**(5):855-859

[100] Cholkar K, Vadlapudi AD, Trinh HM, Mitra AK. Compositions, formulation, pharmacology, pharmacokinetics, and toxicity of topical, periocular, and intravitreal ophthalmic drugs. In: Gilger CB, editor. Ocular Pharmacology and Toxicology. Totowa, N.J: Humana Press; 2014. pp. 91-118

[101] Yang Y, Bailey C, Loewenstein A, Massin P. Intravitreal corticosteroids in diabetic macular edema: Pharmacokinetic considerations. Retina. 2015;**35**(12):2440-2449

[102] Augustin A. Anecortave acetate in the treatment of age-related macular degeneration. Clinical Interventions in Aging. 2006;**3**:237-246

[103] Edelhauser HF, Rendleman CL, Robinson MR, Dawson DG, Chader GJ, Grossniklaus HE. Ophthalmic drug delivery systems for the treatment of retinal diseases: Basic research to clinical applications. Investigative Ophthalmology & Visual Science. 2010;**51**(11):5403-5420

[104] Hayden BC, Jockovich ME, Murray TG, Voigt M, Milne P, Kralinger M. Pharmacokinetics of systemic versus focal carboplatin chemotherapy in the rabbit eye: Possible implication in the treatment of retinoblastoma. Investigative Ophthalmology & Visual Science. 2004;**45**(10):3644-3649

[105] Winter U, Buitrago E, Mena HA, Del Sole MJ, Laurent V, Negrotto S, et al. Pharmacokinetics, safety, and efficacy of intravitreal digoxin in preclinical models for retinoblastoma. Investigative Ophthalmology & Visual Science. 2015;**56**(8):4382-4393

[106] Mannermaa E, Vellonen KS, Urtti A. Drug transport in corneal epithelium and blood–retina barrier: Emerging role of transporters in ocular pharmacokinetics. Advanced Drug Delivery Reviews. 2006;**58**(11):1136-1163

[107] Dey S, Gunda S, Mitra AK. Pharmacokinetics of erythromycin in rabbit corneas after single-dose infusion: Role of P-glycoprotein as a barrier to in vivo ocular drug absorption. Journal of Pharmacology and Experimental Therapeutics. 2004;**311**(1):246-255

[108] Hariharan S, Gunda S, Mishra GP, Pal D, Mitra AK. Enhanced corneal absorption of erythromycin by modulating P-glycoprotein and MRP mediated efflux with corticosteroids. Pharmaceutical Research. 2009;**26**(5): 1270-1282

[109] Hariharan S, Minocha M, Mishra GP, Pal D, Krishna R, Mitra AK. Interaction of ocular hypotensive agents (PGF2α analogs—bimatoprost, latanoprost, and travoprost) with MDR efflux pumps on the rabbit cornea. Journal of Ocular Pharmacology and Therapeutics. 2009;**25**(6):487-498

[110] Majumdar S, Hingorani T, Srirangam R, Gadepalli RS, Rimoldi JM, Repka MA. Transcorneal permeation of L-and D-aspartate ester prodrugs of acyclovir: Delineation of passive diffusion versus transporter involvement. Pharmaceutical Research. 2009;**26**(5):1261-1269

[111] Anand B, Katragadda S, Nashed Y, Mitra A. Amino acid prodrugs of acyclovir as possible

antiviral agents against ocular HSV-1 infections: Interactions with the neutral and cationic amino acid transporter on the corneal epithelium. Current Eye Research. 2004;**29**(2-3):153-166

[112] Jain-Vakkalagadda B, Pal D, Gunda S, Nashed Y, Ganapathy V, Mitra AK. Identification of a Na+–dependent cationic and neutral amino acid transporter, B0,+, in human and rabbit cornea. Molecular Pharmaceutics. 2004;**1**(5):338-346

[113] Anand BS, Mitra AK. Mechanism of corneal permeation of L-valyl ester of acyclovir: Targeting the oligopeptide transporter on the rabbit cornea. Pharmaceutical Research. 2002;**19**(8):1194-1202

[114] Gunda S, Hariharan S, Mitra AK. Corneal absorption and anterior chamber pharmacokinetics of dipeptide monoester prodrugs of ganciclovir (GCV): In vivo comparative evaluation of these prodrugs with Val-GCV and GCV in rabbits. Journal of Ocular Pharmacology & Therapeutics. 2006;**22**(6):465-476

[115] Majumdar S, Nashed YE, Patel K, Jain R, Itahashi M, Neumann DM, et al. Dipeptide monoester ganciclovirprodrugs for treating HSV-1-induced corneal epithelial and stromal keratitis: In vitro and in vivo evaluations. Journal of Ocular Pharmacology & Therapeutics. 2005;**21**(6):463-474

[116] Katragadda S, Talluri RS, Mitra AK. Modulation of P-glycoprotein–mediated efflux by prodrugderivatization: An approach involving peptide transporter–mediated influx across rabbit cornea. Journal of Ocular Pharmacology & Therapeutics. 2006;**22**(2):110-120

[117] Kansara V, Hao Y, Mitra AK. Dipeptide monoester ganciclovirprodrugs for transscleral drug delivery: Targeting the oligopeptide transporter on rabbit retina. Journal of Ocular Pharmacology and Therapeutics. 2007;**23**(4):321-334

[118] Janoria KG, Boddu SH, Wang Z, Paturi DK, Samanta S, Pal D, et al. Vitreal pharmacokinetics of biotinylated-ganciclovir: Role of sodium-dependent multivitamin transporter expressed on retina. Journal of Ocular Pharmacology and Therapeutics. 2009;**25**(1):39-49

[119] Vadlapudi AD, Vadlapatla RK, Earla R, Sirimulla S, Bailey JB, Pal D, et al. Novel biotinylated lipid prodrugs of acyclovir for the treatment of herpetic keratitis (HK): Transporter recognition, tissue stability and antiviral activity. Pharmaceutical Research. 2013;**30**(8):2063-2076

[120] Mandal A, Agrahari V, Khurana V, Pal D, Mitra AK. Transporter effects on cell permeability in drug delivery. Expert Opinion on Drug Delivery. 2017;**14**(3):385-401

[121] Vellonen KS, Soini EM, Del Amo EM, Urtti A. Prediction of ocular drug distribution from systemic blood circulation. Molecular Pharmaceutics. 2016;**13**(9):2906-2911

[122] Boddu SH, Gunda S, Earla R, Mitra AK. Ocular microdialysis: A continuous sampling technique to study pharmacokinetics and pharmacodynamics in the eye. Bioanalysis. 2010;**2**(3):487-507

[123] Danesh-Meyer HV, Zhang J, Acosta ML, Rupenthal ID, Green CR. Connexin43 in retinal injury and disease. Progress in Retinal and Eye Research. 2016;**51**:41-68

[124] Kang-Mieler JJ, Rudeen KM, Liu W, Mieler WF. Advances in ocular drug delivery systems. Eye. 2020;**34**(8):1371-1379

[125] Michael IP. Development of Novel Antiangiogenic Biologics. Canada: University of Toronto; 2011

[126] Cholkar K, Dasari SR, Pal D, Mitra AK. Eye: Anatomy, physiology and barriers to drug delivery. In: Ocular Transporters and Receptors. Woodhead Publishing; 2013. pp. 1-36

[127] Cholkar K, Trinh HM, Vadlapudi AD, Wang Z, Pal D, Mitra AK. Interaction studies of resolvin E1 analog (RX-10045) with efflux transporters. Journal of Ocular Pharmacology and Therapeutics. 2015;**31**(4):248-255

[128] Juuti-Uusitalo K, Vaajasaari H, Ryhänen T, Narkilahti S, Suuronen R, Mannermaa E, et al. Efflux protein expression in human stem cell-derived retinal pigment epithelial cells. PLoS One. 2012;7(1):e30089

[129] Mannermaa E, Vellonen KS, Ryhänen T, Kokkonen K, Ranta VP, Kaarniranta K, et al. Efflux protein expression in human retinal pigment epithelium cell lines. Pharmaceutical Research. 2009;**26**(7):1785-1791

[130] Shah R, Amador C, Tormanen K, Ghiam S, Saghizadeh M, Arumugaswami V, et al. Systemic diseases and the cornea. Experimental Eye Research. 2021;**204**:108455

[131] Sánchez-López E, Espina M, Doktorovova S, Souto EB, García ML. Lipid nanoparticles (SLN, NLC): Overcoming the anatomical and physiological barriers of the eye—Part I—Barriers and determining factors in ocular delivery. European Journal of Pharmaceutics and Biopharmaceutics. 2017;**110**:70-75

[132] Bhujbal SS, Wale KK, Mahale NB, Landage AD, Sayyed SF, Chaudhari SR. Ocular drug delivery system: A review. World Journal of Pharmaceutical Research, RamaiyanDhanapal. 2014;**3**:320-343

[133] Chien YW. Ocular drug delivery and delivery systems. In: Novel Drug Delivery Systems. Vol. 2nd ed. New York: Marcel Dekker; 1992. pp. 269-270

[134] Saettone MF, Salminen L. Ocular inserts for topical delivery. Advance Drug Delivery Review. 1995;**16**:95-106

[135] Khar RK, Vyas SP. Targeted and Controlled Drug Delivery Novel Carrier Systems. New Delhi: CBS Publishers and Distributors; 2002. p. 384

Section 4

In Silico Drug Development

Chapter 5

Computer-Aided Drug Design and Development: An Integrated Approach

Neelima Dhingra

Abstract

Drug discovery and development is a very time- and resource-consuming process. Comprehensive knowledge of chemistry has been integrated with information technology to streamline drug discovery, design, development, and optimization. Computer-aided drug design is being utilized to expedite and facilitate hit identification, hit-to-lead selection, and optimize the absorption, distribution, metabolism, excretion, and toxicity profile. Regulatory organizations and the pharmaceutical industry are continuously involved in the development of computational techniques that will improve the effectiveness and efficiency of the drug discovery process while decreasing the use of animals, cost, and time and increasing predictability. The present chapter will provide an overview of computational tools, such as structure-based and receptor-based drug designing, and how the coupling of these tools with a rational drug design process has led to the discovery of small molecules as therapeutic agents for numerous human disease conditions duly approved by the Food and Drug Administration. It is expected that the power of CADD will grow as the technology continues to evolve.

Keywords: drug discovery, Cheminformatics, CADD, success stories

1. Introduction

> *"This is a fantastic time to be doing drug discovery. We have an incredible wealth of knowledge that has been generated over the past few years."*

Drug discovery and development (DD&D) is a lengthy and complex process that takes around 12–15 years and costs up to multi-million dollars for a drug to reach the market. Interdisciplinary DD&D begins with the identification and validation of a suitable drug target, followed by a hit to lead discovery and optimization, and finally preclinical and clinical studies. Despite the huge investments and time incurred for the discovery of new drugs, the success rates are too low that only five out of 10,000 compounds make their way to reach human testing after preliminary evaluation in animals and only one of five compounds reaches final clinical studies. Further, a majority (40–60%) of the drug failure has been observed at a later stage of the DD&D process due to a lack of optimal pharmacokinetic properties, that is, absorption, distribution, metabolism, excretion, and toxicity (ADME/Tox). This all suggested and urged the need to develop new methodologies to facilitate and expedite the DD&D process [1].

Advances in computational techniques and parallel hardware support have enabled computer-aided drug design (*in silico*) methods, that are being used by leading pharmaceutical companies and research groups to speed up the DD&D process. It entails:

- Usage of computing power to simplify drug discovery and development process
- Leveraging the chemical and biological information about targets and/or ligands to identify and optimize new drugs
- Designing *in silico* filters to remove compounds with poor activity and/or poor ADMET
- Selection of the most promising candidates.

Broadly classified computational methods include combinatorial chemistry; high throughput screening; virtual screening; pharmacophore modeling structure-based drug design (drug-target docking); ligand-based drug design (pharmacophore, a 3-D spatial arrangement of chemical features essential for biological activity)—quantitative structure-activity and structure-property relationships; quantum mechanics and *in silico* evaluation methods [2]. The commonly and widely used CADD approaches are structure-based and ligand-based drug design approaches, to identify suitable lead molecules in the drug discovery process. The structure-based drug design (SBDD) relies on the three-dimensional (3D) structure of the target receptor and its active sites to understand the molecular interaction between the receptor and ligand. While the ligand-based-drug design (LBDD) depends on the knowledge of ligands interacting with the given target receptor. A few marginally active or better compounds may be found, and then chemical similarity searching techniques are used to find more compounds that can be assayed. Finding some of the more active compounds further computationally techniques are applied to identify more potent compounds with favorable ADME/T [2, 3].

The application of rational drug design as an integral part of CADD provides useful insights into the understanding of the binding affinity and molecular interaction between target and ligand. Additionally, lead identification in pharmaceutical research has been facilitated by the availability of the super-computing facility, parallel processing, and advanced programs, algorithms, and tools. Furthermore, recent advancements in artificial intelligence (AI) and machine learning methods have greatly aided in analyzing, learning, and explaining the pharmaceutical-related big data in the drug discovery process [4].

2. Structure-based drug design

2.1 Docking

Understanding the principles by which small-molecule (ligands) recognize and interact with a receptor (macromolecules target) is of great importance in the

Simulation approach	Shape complementarity approach
Interaction energy as per ligand-receptor pair is calculated.	Estimation of complementarity between ligand and receptor surface.
Ligand is allowed to fit into the receptor's groove based upon minimum energy consideration.	Solvent accessible topographic features of ligand and receptor in terms of matching surface are described.
Every move of ligand into receptor's pocket for best fitting generates energy as Total Energy of System and is compared to find out best-docked conformer with minimum energy.	It involves the surface representation of receptor and ligand (i.e., surface construction and smoothing), features/curvature calculation followed by docking and scoring contingent on geometric complementary criteria.
More compatible to accept ligand flexibility in the molecular modeling tool.	Both types of docking; flexible docking and rigid docking are feasible.
Requires much longer time as large energy profiling needs to be estimated.	Rapid scanning of a large number of ligands for the binding on its target in a few seconds and hence provides quick and robust outcomes.

Table 1.
Molecular docking approaches.

pharmaceutical research and development (R&D) process. The availability and systematic use of the three-dimensional (3D) structure of the therapeutic target proteins and exploration of the binding site cavity form the basis of structure-based drug design (SBDD). This specific and fast approach identifies the lead molecules followed by their optimization and helps to understand disease at a molecular level. Some of the common methods employed in SBDD include structure-based virtual screening (SBVS), molecular docking, and molecular dynamics (MD) simulations. In case of the non-availability of structural information of the desired target, another computational approach, that is, homology modeling can be utilized to build the model of the needed target [5].

Molecular docking is one of the most commonly used techniques in SBDD, because of its ability to predict with a significant degree of accuracy the conformation of small-molecule ligands within the applicable target binding site. Two approaches are primarily used to perform molecular docking, the simulation approach, and the shape complimentary approach. The first approach utilizes computer simulations wherein the energy profiling is assessed for ligand-target docked conformer. Whereas, the second approach employs the practice that calculates surface complementarity between ligand and target. The brief and main properties of both approaches are described in **Table 1** [6].

2.2 Methodology

It is a cyclic process with basic steps of the preparation of target structure, binding site prediction, ligand preparation using generated library of synthesized compounds, molecular docking, binding free energy calculations, analysis based on these scoring functions, and molecular dynamic simulation. In the last few decades, advancement in structural elucidation techniques, such as X-ray and NMR, has increased the availability of protein structure deposits in protein data bank (PDB). However, some of the target protein structures have not been solved to date and computational techniques, such as comparative homology modeling, ab initio modeling and threading are successful in interpreting the structures of such proteins from their sequences. After the target selection, it's important to identify the ligand-binding site, a prerequisite step for carrying out specific docking. The information on the binding sites can be obtained from the X-ray crystallographic structures of proteins co-crystallized with substrates or inhibitors or through site-directed mutagenesis study. In the absence of the experimental information about the binding site of many proteins, plenty of software and webservers such DoGSite Scorer, CASTp, DEPTH, and NSiteMatch, allows us to predict the putative binding sites of the isolated and purified protein [7]. For a particular selected prepared protein, a library of the compounds retrieved from chemical databases, ZINC database, DrugBank, PubChem, or synthesized molecules in the research laboratories can be tested. Also, it preferred to perform the docking on drug-like compounds being filtered using Lipinski's rule of five and ADMET (absorption, distribution, metabolism, excretion, and toxicity) parameters, including risk parameters, such as acute rat toxicity, carcinogenicity, hepatotoxicity, and mutagenicity [8].

2.3 Interpretation and correlation

The ultimate purpose of the SBDD is to visualize ligands with specific electrostatic (charge distribution) and stereochemical (bulky or small) attributes to achieve high receptor-binding affinity. First, developed algorithms for molecular docking in 1980, enabled us to understand crucial molecular events, such as ligand-binding modes and their corresponding intermolecular interactions that stabilize the ligand-receptor complex [9]. The availability of 3D protein (macromolecular) structures further facilitated a careful inspection of the binding site topology, as well as the presence of cavities, clefts, and sub-pockets. Investigations arrange and rank the docked compounds based on the specific scoring functions of ligand-receptor complexes after quantitative predictions of their binding energetics [9]. Molecular docking programs identify the most likely binding conformations after cyclical steps of exploring the large conformational space representing various potential binding modes and accurate prediction of the interaction energy coupled with each of these predicted binding conformations [10].

These molecular modeling procedures are followed by the synthesis of the most promising compounds, and their biological properties evaluations using diverse *in vitro* and *in vivo* experimental protocols. Once the active compounds have been identified, the 3D structures of such ligand-receptor complexes from docking studies allow the observation of numerous intermolecular features supporting the process of molecular recognition. Structural descriptions of these complexes are helpful in investigating the binding conformations, key intermolecular interactions, characterization of unknown binding sites, mechanistic studies, and the elucidation of ligand-induced conformational changes [11]. Then biological activity data can be justified and correlated to structural information once a ligand-receptor complex has been determined.

In this way, the SBDD process in CADD starts over with new steps to design ligand by incorporating necessary molecular modifications for efficient or increased affinity toward the binding site. And selective adjustments of a validated drug target by high-affinity ligands ultimately lead to the desired pharmacological and therapeutic effects by interfering with specific cellular processes. The flexibility of the target receptor always remains an essential aspect to be considered throughout the modeling phase, as substantial conformational changes can occur upon its binding with the ligand. To address the issue, two modified approaches flexible docking (flexible-ligand and flexible-protein search docking) and molecular dynamics were further tried and

S. No.	Software tools	Algorithm	Scoring term	Advantages
1.	Glide	Monte Carlo	Glide score	Lead discovery and lead optimization
2.	AutoDock	Lamarckian genetic algorithm	Empirical free energy function	Adaptability to user-defined input
3.	GOLD	Genetic algorithm	GoldScore, ChemScore, ASP CHEMPLP	Allows atomic overlapping between protein and ligand
4.	ICM	Monte Carlo minimization	Virtual library screening scoring function	Allows side-chain flexibility to find a parallel arrangement of two rigid helixes

Table 2.
List of software tools for docking and their algorithms [14].

explored. Stochastic method, systematic method, and simulation method are the three commonly used algorithms for ligand flexibility in the case of the flexible-ligand search docking method, whereas flexible-protein docking usually depends on molecular dynamic (MD) and Monte Carlo (MC) methods [12].

2.4 Application and tools

SBDD as a computational technique has greatly helped many pharmaceutical industries and medicinal chemists in the discovery of several drugs available on the market. Few of them include the discovery of amprenavir as a potential inhibitor of the human immune deficiency virus (HIV) protease using homology protein modeling and MD simulations; norfloxacin a commonly used antibiotic against urinary tract infection using SBVS, isoniazid (antituberculosis drug) an enoyl-acyl-ACP reductase (InhA) inhibitor discovered through SBVS and pharmacophore modeling, and flurbiprofen, a nonsteroidal anti-inflammatory (NSAID) drug used against rheumatoid and osteoarthritis targeting cyclooxygenase-2 (COX-2) discovered through molecular docking approach, etc. [13]. Some of the freely available software tools for docking study are enlisted in **Table 2** summarizing their algorithms, scoring functions, and advantages.

3. Ligand-based drug design

Ligand-based drug design is an extensively used approach in computer-aided drug designing, especially when the three-dimensional structure of the target receptor is not available. The information derived from a set of active compounds against a particular target receptor can be used in the identification of structural and physicochemical properties accountable for the given biological activity, based on the fact that structural resemblances correspond to similar biological functions. Pharmacophore modeling [15] and quantitative structure-activity relationships (QSARs) [16] are some of the conventional techniques used in ligand-based virtual screening (LBVS).

Generated pharmacophore model elucidates the spatial arrangement of chemical features in ligands that are essential for interaction with the target receptor. H-bond donors/acceptors, hydrophobic areas, aromatic ring systems, and +ve/−ve charged ionizable groups are some of the chemical features used in pharmacophore modeling.

Ligands with different scaffolds but the similar spatial arrangement of the above-mentioned key interacting functional moieties can be identified using pharmacophore-based virtual screening [15]. The conformation of the active molecules within the target binding site can be integrated into the pharmacophore model for further application in QSAR studies in the molecular alignment stage.

3.1 Quantitative structure-activity relationships (QSARs)

Quantitative structure-activity relationship (QSAR) analysis is the most commonly utilized LBDD approach and correlates the variations in the bioactivity of the compounds with the changes in molecular structure. A statistically significant model is being constructed using these correlation studies, and the final model can be utilized to predict the biological activity of new molecules [17]. They are widely used in the drug discovery process in the hit to lead identification or lead optimization.

The technique was developed more than 50 years ago by Hansch and Fujita (1964), where affinities of ligands to their binding sites, rate, and inhibition constants were correlated with other biological endpoints with the atomic, group, or molecular properties, such as lipophilicity, electronic parameters, polarizability, and steric properties (Hansch analysis), or with some structural features (Free-Wilson analysis) [18]. But, the limitation of the classical approach in designing a new molecule on account of the lack of understanding of the 3D structure of the molecules urged the scientists to look for an alternative. So, an extension to the existing classical Hansch and Free-Wilson approaches emerged as 3D-QSAR, which exploits the three-dimensional properties of the ligands to predict their biological activities. Since then and until now, QSAR continues an efficient approach for building mathematical models to find a statistically significant correlation between the chemical structure and continuous (pIC_{50}, pEC_{50}, Ki, etc.) or categorical/binary (active, inactive, toxic, nontoxic, etc.) biological/toxicological property using regression and classification techniques, respectively [19].

In the last decades, QSAR has undergone several transformations, ranging from the dimensionality of the molecular descriptors (**Table 3**) and different methods (**Table 4**) for finding a correlation between the chemical structures and the biological property. Based on how the descriptors are derived, QSAR can be classified into six different types (**Table 5**) [20].

Depending on the quantity of dataset, QSARs can be classified and designed as local or global. A local QSAR is trained on a small and congeneric series of chemical structures, whereas a large and structurally diverse set of chemicals are used for

Hydrophobic descriptors	Partition coefficient, Hansch's substitution constant, distribution coefficient, hydrophobic fragmental constant, solubility parameter
Electronic descriptors	Hammett constant, Taft's inductive (polar) constant, ionization constant, Swain and Lupton field parameter
Steric descriptors	Taft's steric parameter, Vander Walls volume, molar volume, molar refractivity, and Vander Walls radius.
Spatial descriptors	Shadow indices, principle moment of inertia, the radius of gyration
Quantum chemical descriptors	Atomic net charge, super delocalizability, energy of lowest unoccupied molecular orbital. The energy of the highest occupied molecular orbital

Table 3.
Types of descriptors in different QSAR.

Linear method	Linear regression (LR), multiple linear regression (MLR), partial least squares (PLS), principal component analysis (PCA), and principal component regression (PCR).
Nonlinear	k-nearest neighbors (kNN), artificial neural networks (ANN), and Bayesian neural nets [20].

Table 4.
QSAR classification based on the methodology.

One dimensional (1D)	Correlates the activity with global molecular properties, such as pKa and log P
Two (2) dimensional	Correlates the activity with structural patterns, such as connectivity indices, and 2D pharmacophore without considering the 3D representation of these properties
Three (3) dimensional	Activity is correlated with noncovalent interaction fields surrounding the molecules
Four (4) dimensional	It further includes set of ligand configurations in 3D QSAR.
Five (5) dimensional	Explicitly represents the different induced fit models in 4D QSAR.
Six(6) dimensional 6D	Additionally, it incorporates the solvation models in 5D QSAR

Table 5.
QSAR classification based on parameter correlated.

global QSAR [21]. The development of the QSAR model follows a general workflow as shown in **Figure 1**, starting from the collection of the dataset, its curation, and preparation, followed by the generation and selection of chemical descriptors to be used as independent variables. Collected data is divided into training and test sets, and the QSAR model is built using a training set consisting of chemical structures and their related experimental data. The chemical structures are represented by chemical descriptors, which are used as independent variables in the model. Statistically significant model (s) are built within the defined applicability domains (AD) based on field-based or atom-based approaches. In field QSAR, the molecule atoms are treated as fields and classified as either H-bond acceptor, H-bond donor, electrostatic or stearic. On the other hand, in atom-based QSAR, molecule atoms are considered spheres and can predict the results for H-bond donor/acceptor, non-polar/hydrophobic, negative/positive ionic, or electron-withdrawing groups. Both methods can predict the change in activity by the fields or spheres in molecules with various types of substitution [22].

Validation is the process to access the reliability and relevance of a particular approach, method, or process established for a defined purpose. Certainly, it is possible to calculate a large number of descriptors using various software tools, however, one cannot ignore the risk of chance correlations with the higher number of variables incorporated in the final model as compared to the number of compounds for which the model has been constructed. And with diverse optimization procedures, one can try to get models that can fit the experimental data well, but there is always a chance of overfitting. Thus, all indicate the necessity to validate the developed models for their robustness and predictivity. And QSAR models are fundamentally judged for their predictivity, which represents how well they are capable to forecast the end-point values of molecules being not employed to develop the correlation. QSAR models can be validated using two major strategies: (i) internal validation based on the training set molecules, and (ii) external validation using the test set compounds after splitting the whole data set into training and test sets. Validation and analysis are characterized in terms of statistical parameters, such as regression values (R2),

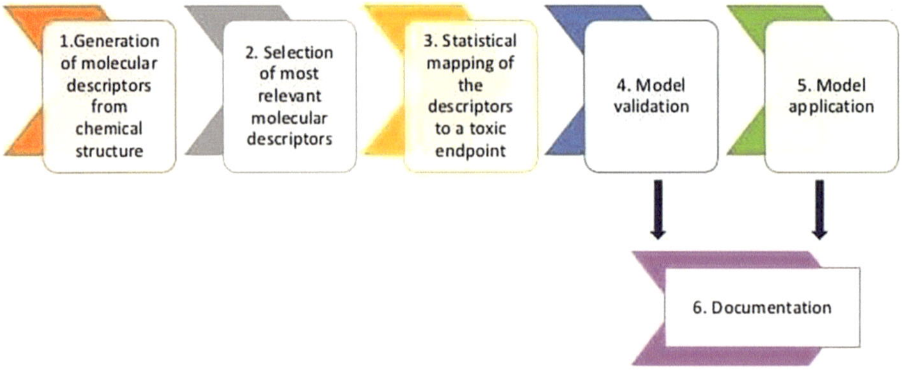

Figure 1.
Workflow of ligand based drug designing.

variance ratios (F), standard deviations (SD), root mean square error of the test set (RMSE), anticipated activities of the test set (Q2), and Pearson-R, were used to validate and analyze the model generated [18].

3.2 Tools

Quantitative structure-activity relationships (QSAR) have been applied for decades in the development of new drugs. Although a QSAR does not completely eliminate the trial-and-error factor involved in the development of a new drug, it

Software	Description	Availability
ACD/Tox Suite	Prediction of toxicity	Commercial, free web service
ADMET Predictor	ADMET properties prediction	Commercial
AZ Orange Machine learning platform for	QSAR modeling	Free
3D-QSAR	3D QSAR models	Free
BioTriangle	Web-based platform to calculate the molecular descriptors	Free
BioPPsy	Prediction of pharmacokinetic properties of drug candidates by QSPR modeling	Free
BlueDesc	Molecular Descriptor Calculator	Free
CAESAR	Developments of toxicity models	Free
CACTVS	Molecular descriptor calculator	Free
CODESSA	Generate predictive QSAR models from quantum chemical, topological and electrostatic descriptors	Commercial
ChemDes	Calculations of descriptor and fingerprint (web-based)	Free

Table 6.
Software's and their features [14].

certainly decreases the number of compounds synthesized by facilitating the selection of the most promising examples. A number of successful QSAR studies have been carried out using various platforms and helped in building models for predicting chemical, biological and toxicological activities. Some of these are listed in **Table 6**.

4. In silico 5-AlPHA reductase activity prediction using SBDD

Benign prostatic hyperplasia (BPH), a common condition of males over the age of 50 is characterized by enlargement of the prostate and results in urinary obstructions. Dihydrotestosterone (DHT), the 5α-reduced metabolite of testosterone (T) (**Figure 2**) has been implicated as a causative factor in this progression of BPH. 5-alpha reductase (5AR) a membrane-bound NADPH-dependent enzyme is responsible for the irreversible conversion of androgen T into DHT in the prostate. And inhibition of 5AR represents a logical treatment for controlling the BPH by diminishing the concentration of DHT in the prostate and is expected to improve the pathology of this disease [23].

In the past few decades, numerous nonsteroidal and steroidal compounds have been prepared as competitive or noncompetitive inhibitors of 5AR [24, 25]. In 1992,

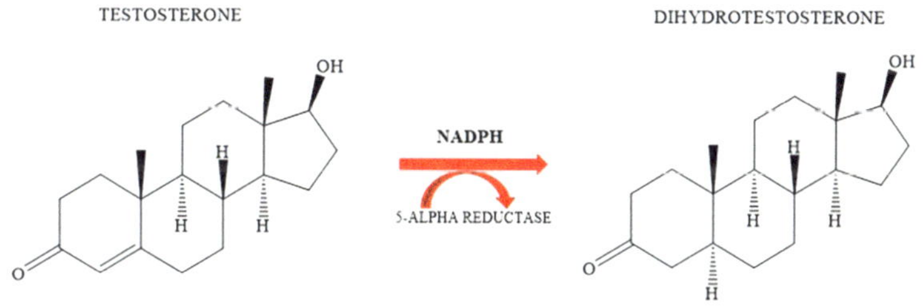

Figure 2.
Action of 5-alpha reductase (5AR).

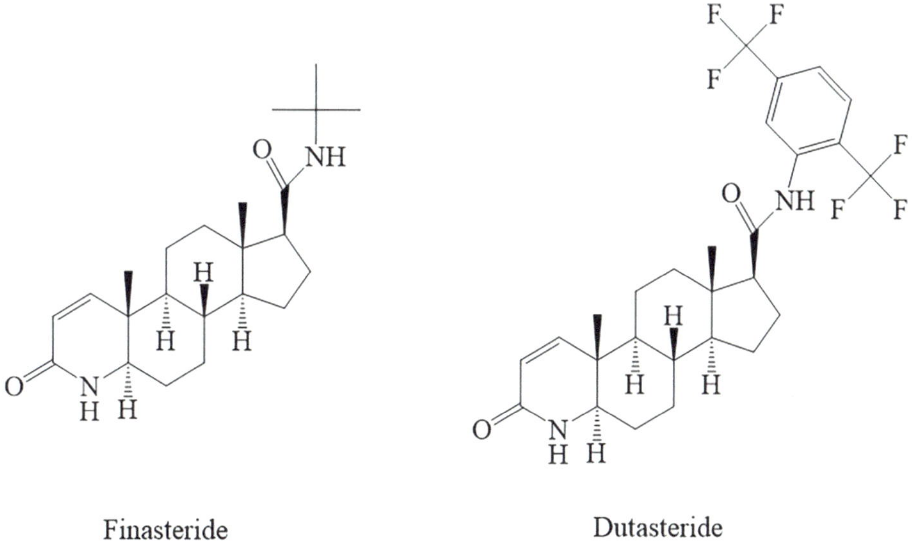

Figure 3.
Clinically approved 5-alpha reductase inhibitors.

Finasteride (MK-906) was approved as the first 5-alpha reductase inhibitor (5ARI) in the United States for the clinical management of BPH. It is a competitive inhibitor of 5AR type-2 and at the clinical doses of 5 mg/day, it forms a stable complex with a 10-fold higher affinity than type 1 and decreases the prostatic DHT level and prostate volume by 70–90%, in human beings. Unlike finasteride, another molecule, that is,

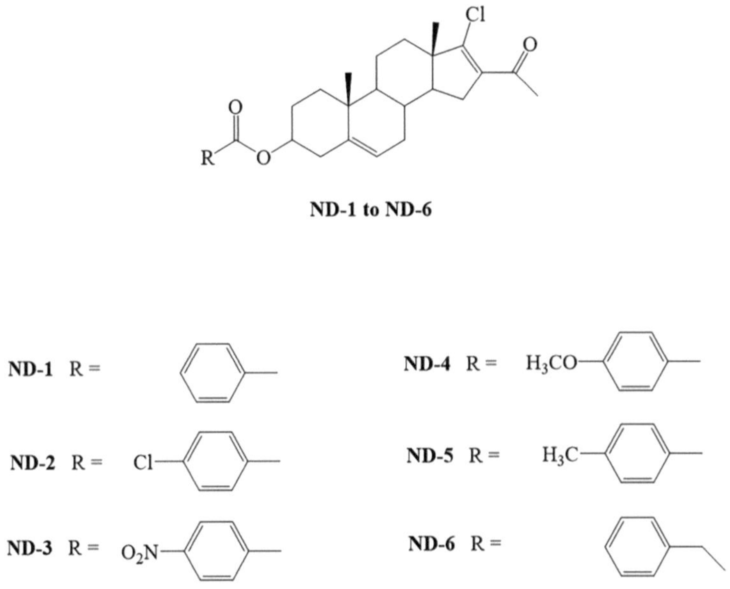

Figure 4.
Novel 5-alpha reductase inhibitors synthesized in our laboratory.

S. No.	Compounds	D-score	No. of residues	Hydrophobic	Aromatic	Hydrogen
1	*ND-1*	−66.23	5	ALA60A, ALA59A, ILE31A, SER471A, ALA32A	—	—
2	*ND-2*	−62.87	6	ALA59A, ALA292A, THR175A, ALA264A, THRS60A, LEU472A	—	—
3	*ND-3*	−74.91	7	ALA59A, ALA63A, THRS175A, THRS60A	—	GLY241A, GLY245A
4	*ND-4*	−60.68	8	ALA63A, ALA59A, THRS175A, ILE31A, SER471A, ALA32A, GLY30A	—	GLY310A
5	*ND-5*	−59.75	8	ALA63A, ALA59A, ALA264A, ALA45A, LEU472A, GLY475A, ALA32A, GLY455A	—	—
6	*ND-6*	−62.79	6	ALA59A, THR175A, ALA63A, SER471A, ALA264A	HIS268A	—
7	FN	−57.09	10	GLY176A, LEU62A, ALA59A, SER471A, ILE31A, LEU472A, GLY475A, GLY455A, ARG456A, THR175A	—	—

Table 7.
Docking score of novel 5ARIs.

dutasteride (**Figure 3**) a nonselective competitive inhibitor of both isozymes. 5AR type-1 and type-2 were approved in 2002 by the USA for the symptomatic treatment of BPH [26].

Since then, only finasteride and dutasteride are being used, but their long-term treatment has been found to be associated with the development of decreased libido, impotence or ejaculatory dysfunction, or, breast enlargement while rashes, insulin resistance, type 2 diabetes, kidney dysfunction, and other metabolic dysfunctions [26]. Thus, the identification of highly efficacious and selective inhibitors of 5AR for use in the treatment of BPH has engendered considerable interest from research groups in several laboratories. Attempts have been made in our laboratory to synthesize and characterize novel 5ARIs (**ND-1 to ND-6**) (**Figure 4**).

Structure-based drug designing approach, that is, docking (*in silico*) was performed on the newly synthesized compounds (**ND-1 to ND-6**) against PDBID: 4AT0 of 5AR receptor, using extra precision GRIP docking feature in BIOPREDICTA module available in the molecular design suite of Vlife MDS software package, version 4.6. Reference drug finasteride (FN) known to possess an affinity for the 5AR receptor was also included in the docking studies for comparing the docking results. Studies have shown that all the synthesized compounds have been found to bound better with

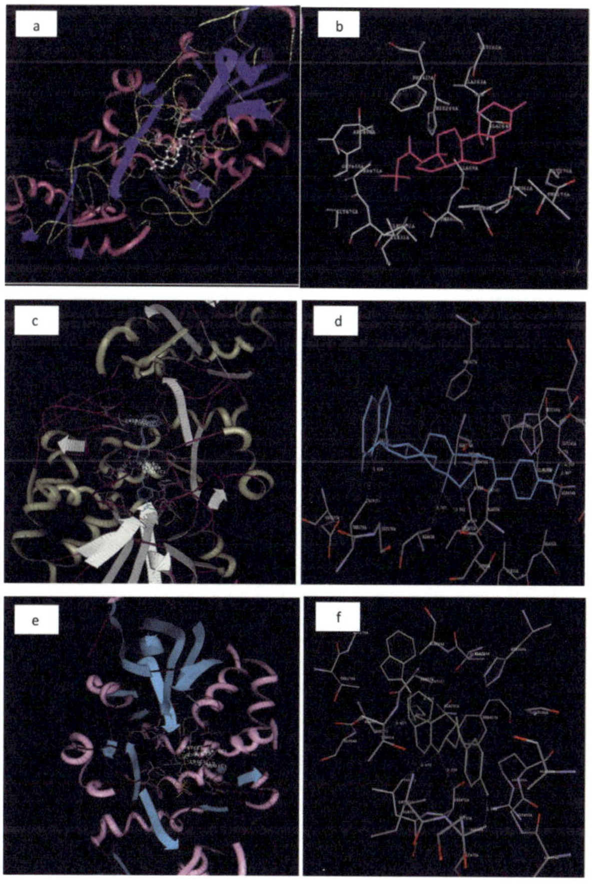

Figure 5.
(a, c, and e) Grip docked pose of standard drug FN, ND-1, and ND 3 into the active binding site of 5AR receptor; (b, d, and f) 2D representation of the FN, ND-1, and ND 3 with active amino residues of 5AR receptor.

the 5AR receptor affording dock score from −59.75 to −74.91 than reference, finasteride −57.09 (**Table 7**).

The docking score has been observed in order ND3 > ND1 > ND2 > ND6 > ND4 and ND5. Further, similar docking behavior has been observed among all the synthesized compounds in comparison to FN, by interacting hydrophobically with common amino acid residues THR175A, ALA59A, ALA63A, SER471A, and ALA264A. Additional aromatic interactions have also been observed only in ND-6 for amino acid HIS268A. Among all the newly synthesized derivatives ND-1 to ND-6, **ND-3** has been found to bound best with the 5AR receptor affording the highest D-score of −74.91 than FN. This high score of −74.91 can be attributed to its strong hydrogen bonds between NO_2 at the p-position of the benzene ring with amino acid residue GLY241A and GLY245A. The binding pose of the fitted ligands was visualized extending deep into the active site pocket and are presented in the **Figure 5a–f**.

5. Conclusion

In the pharmaceutical industries, Research and Development is undergoing a lot of technological changes, and there is pressure to make the investment pay off. There is a massive demand to sensibly use the big amount of chemical and biological-related data produced in the process. Careful use of chemoinformatics techniques and software is becoming crucial in drug discovery success and an evolving field with many facets. In the past few years, it has led to the discovery of small-molecule therapeutic agents with activity directed against target proteins critical in the presentation of numerous disease conditions and/or have supported their clinical evaluation. Coupling more sophisticated computer software and hardware technologies with a rational drug design process has become an indispensable tool for the development of effective therapies and it yields information that is not easy to obtain in laboratory analysis, and, furthermore, is typically (much) less costly, save time, money, and resources. It is expected that the power of CADD will grow as the technology continues to evolve.

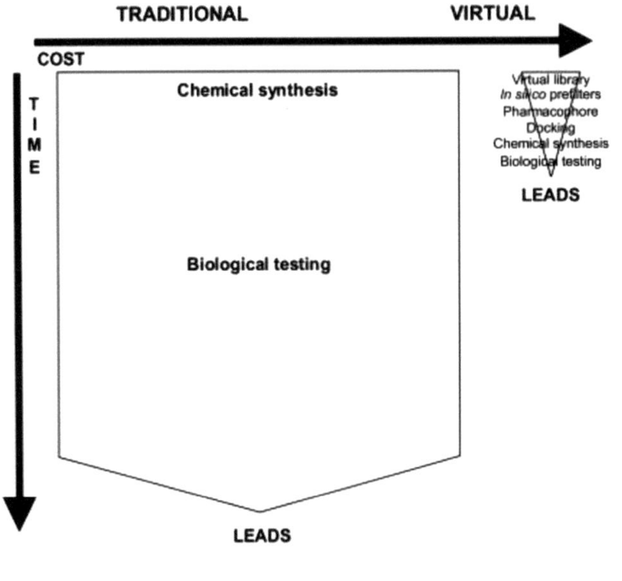

Author details

Neelima Dhingra
University Institute of Pharmaceutical Sciences, Panjab University, Chandigarh, India

*Address all correspondence to: neelimad08@gmail.com

References

[1] Usha T, Shanmugarajan D, Goyal AK, Kumar CS, Middha SK. Recent updates on computer-aided drug discovery: Time for a paradigm shift. Current Topics in Medicinal Chemistry. 2017;**17**(30):3296-3307

[2] Kiriiri GK, Njogu PM, Mwangi AN. Exploring different approaches to improve the success of drug discovery and development projects: A review. Future Journal of Pharmaceutical Sciences. 2020;**6**(1):27-39

[3] de Souza Ribeiro M, de Carvalho LN. Role of computer aided drug design in drug development and drug discovery. Angewandte Chemie International Edition. 2000;**6**(11):951-952

[4] Sliwoski G, Kothiwale S, Meiler J, Lowe EW. Computational methods in drug discovery. Pharmacological Reviews. 2014;**66**:334-395

[5] Sharma B, Sharma S. Computer aided drug design: A promising approach for drug discovery. IJCA Proceedings on National Conference on Advances in Computing Applications NCACA. 2016;**1**:1-3

[6] Chaudhary KK, Mishra N. A review on molecular docking: Novel tool for drug discovery. JSM Chemistry. 2016;**4**(3):1029-1032

[7] Singh N, Chaput L, Villoutreix BO. Virtual screening web servers: Designing chemical probes and drug candidates in the cyberspace. Briefings in Bioinformatics. 2021;**22**:1790-1818

[8] Potemkin V, Potemkin A, Grishina M. Internet resources for drug discovery and design. Current Topics in Medicinal Chemistry. 2018;**18**(22):1955-1975

[9] In silico-chemico-biological approach. Chemico-Biological Interactions. 2008;**171**(2):165-176

[10] Grinter SZ, Zou X. Challenges, applications, and recent advances of protein-ligand docking in structure-based drug design. Molecules. 2014;**19**: 10150-10176

[11] Fang Y. Ligand-receptor interaction platforms and their applications for drug discovery. Expert Opinion on Drug Discovery. 2012;7:969-988

[12] Bao C, Subramanian J, Sharma SD. Managing protein flexibility in docking and its applications. Drug Discovery Today. 2009;**14**:394-400

[13] Talele T, Khedkar S, Rigby A. Successful applications of computer aided drug discovery: Moving drugs from concept to the clinic. Current Topics in Medicinal Chemistry. 2010;**10**(1):127-141

[14] Liao C, Sitzmann M, Pugliese A, Nicklaus MC. Software and resources for computational medicinal chemistry. Future Medicinal Chemistry. 2011;**3**:1057-1085

[15] Gao Q, Yang L, Zhu Y. Pharmacophore based drug design approach as a practical process in drug discovery. Current Computer-Aided Drug Design. 2010;**6**(1):37-49

[16] Vrontaki E, Melagraki G, Afantitis A, Tsantili-Kakoulidou A, Mavromoustakos T. 3D quantitative structure–activity relationships (3D-QSAR): A short overview. Pharmakeftiki. 2015;**27**:126-137

[17] Wold S, Johansson E, Cocchi M. PLS - Partial least-squares projections to latent

structures. In: 3D QSAR in Drug Design; Theory, Methods and Applications, Kubinyi H, Editor. Leiden Holland: ESCOM Science Publishers. 1993:523-550

[18] Hansch C, Maloney PP, Fujita T, Muir RM. Correlation of biological activity of phenoxyacetic acids with Hammett substituent constants and partition coefficients. Nature. 1962;**194**(4824):178-180

[19] Cherkasov A, Muratov EN, Fourches D, Varnek A, Baskin II, Cronin M, et al. QSAR modeling: Where have you been? Where are you going to? Journal of Medicinal Chemistry. 2014;**57**: 4977-5010

[20] Alvarez-Ginarte YM, Crespo R, Montero-Cabrera LA, Ruiz-Garcia JA, Ponce YM, Santana R, et al. A novel in-silico approach for QSAR studies of anabolic and androgenic activities in the 17β-hydroxy-5α-androstane steroid family. QSAR and Combinatorial Science. 2005;**24**(2):218-226

[21] Peter SC, Dhanjal JK, Malik V, Radhakrishnan N, Jayakanthan M, Sundar D, et al. Quantitative structure–activity relationship (QSAR): Modeling approaches to biological applications. Encyclopedia of Bioinformatics and Computational Biology: ABC of Bioinformatics. 2019;**1-3**:661-676

[22] Baskin II, Zhokhova NI. The continuous molecular fields approach to building 3D-QSAR models. Journal of Computer-Aided Molecular Design. 2013;**27**(5):427-442

[23] Dhingra N, Bhagwat D. Benign prostatic hyperplasia: An overview of existing treatment. Indian Journal of Pharmacology. 2011;**43**(1):6-12

[24] Alauddin M, Martin-Smith M. Biological activity in steroids possessing nitrogen atoms: Part II. Steroidal alkaloids. Journal of Pharmacy and Pharmacology. 1962;**14**:469-495

[25] Structure–activity relationships for inhibition of 5a-reductase and of androgen receptor binding. Journal of Medicinal Chemistry. 1986;**29**(11):2298-2315

[26] Hirshburg JM, Kelsey PA, Therrien CA, Gavino AC, Reichenberg JS. Adverse effects and safety of 5-alpha reductase inhibitors (finasteride, dutasteride): A systematic review. The Journal of Clinical and Aesthetic Dermatology. 2016;**9**:56-62

Chapter 6

Machine Learning and Artificial Intelligence in Therapeutics and Drug Development Life Cycle

Subhomoi Borkotoky, Amit Joshi, Vikas Kaushik and Anupam Nath Jha

Abstract

In recent years, the pharmaceutical business has seen a considerable increase in data digitization. With digitization, however, comes the challenge of obtaining, analyzing, and applying knowledge to solve complex clinical problems. Artificial intelligence (AI), which entails a variety of advanced tools and networks that can mimic human intellect, can overcome such challenges with traditional pharmaceutical development. Artificial intelligence and machine learning have a vast role in therapeutic development, including the prediction of drug target and properties of small molecules. By predicting the 3D protein structure, AI techniques, such as Alpha Fold, can help with structure-based drug development. Machine learning algorithms have been utilized to anticipate the properties of small molecules based on their chemical structure. Many researches have shown the importance of using *in silico* predictive ADMET (absorption, distribution, metabolism, excretion, and toxicity) models to speed up the discovery of small compounds with enhanced efficacy, safety, and dosage. This chapter discusses various roles of these methods in the development of effective therapeutics.

Keywords: ADMET, deep learning, neural network, virtual screening, QSAR

1. Introduction

The goal of the drug development process is to find bioactive molecules that can help in disease therapy [1, 2]. The drug discovery life cycle has multiple steps: drug target identification, target validation, hit identification, lead optimization, preclinical development, clinical trial, approval, and postmarketing monitoring (**Figure 1A**). Because going through all of these stages of developing a new drug can cost between \$1 and \$2 billion and take 10–17 years, drug discovery is a big issue in the pharmaceutical business [3]. To speed up the drug discovery process, a considerable number of developments were made in the 1990s using combinatorial and high-throughput screening (HTS) approaches. These approaches were widely used since they allowed for the quick synthesis and screening of vast libraries, but no meaningful success was achieved, and little progress was made toward the discovery of new compounds. To

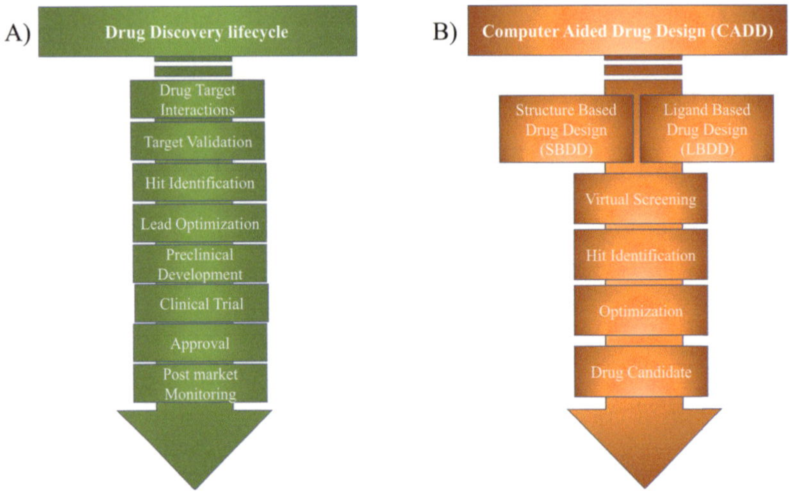

Figure 1.
Flowchart of events taken place in (A) drug discovery lifecycle and (B) computer aided drug discovery.

aid the discovery process, a combination of modern computer approaches, biological research, and chemical synthesis was developed, and this combined approach increased the scope of discovery. The term "computer-aided drug design" (CADD) was eventually used to describe the use of computers in drug discovery. Computer-aided drug design (CADD) is one of the most widely utilized approach for reducing drug development costs and time. CADD is a specialized field, in which various computational approaches are employed to mimic receptor–drug interactions in order to identify binding affinities (**Figure 1B**). The approach, however, is not just for studying chemical interactions and predicting binding affinity; it can be used for everything from designing compounds with desired physiochemical features to managing digital databases of chemicals. CADD is a wide term that encompasses both structure- and ligand-based drug developments. Virtual screening (VS) is a computational method for screening large databases of compounds that has successfully supplemented HTS in drug discovery. The fundamental purpose of VS is to make it feasible to quickly and cheaply screen enormous virtual chemical databases for potential leads for synthesis and future study [4]. Computer-assisted virtual screenings have been a widely used method for estimating various types of ligands to bind with target over time [5–8]. Additionally, in order to investigate atomistic level of protein/nucleic acid-small molecule interactions, one of the widely utilized computational biophysics tools is molecular dynamics (MD) simulation [9, 10]. MD simulation finds its relevance in shedding lights on the conformational ensembles either of the small molecule or of the target. The technique is seldom utilized to capture the dynamics of proteins and/or to check the stability of modeled protein structures enabling CADD for designing efficient inhibitors [11, 12]. It is also leveraged to investigate a comparative binding of small molecule to different proteins along with complementing experimental observations [13].

The recent expansion of make-on-demand libraries to billions of synthesizable molecules has piqued the interest of the drug-discovery community, as such massive databases allow access to previously unexplored chemical realms. The introduction of ultralarge libraries, on the other hand, has revealed substantial limitations of traditional docking techniques, which typically work on the scale of millions of molecules

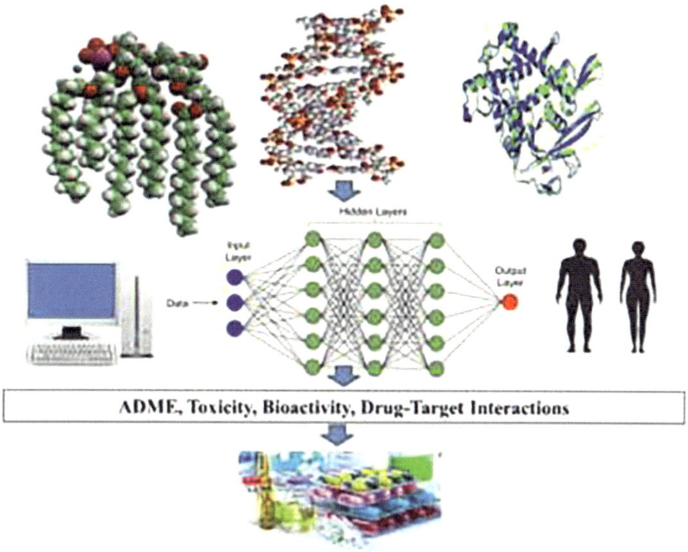

Figure 2.
Biomolecular analysis core scheme for drug discovery via AI/ML.

at a high cost of computation. This aspect depicts CADD as a very useful process, in which only a small portion of the highest-scoring compounds often leaving low scoring but potential compounds are considered for experimental examination. Artificial intelligence (AI) and machine learning (ML) aided approaches provide a low-cost, high-reliability solution to a variety of problems (**Figure 2**), from protein three-dimensional (3D) structure prediction to physiochemical property calculation and bioactivity prediction to ultralarge docking [14, 15].

2. Artificial intelligence (AI) and machine learning (ML)

The ultimate goal of artificial intelligence (AI) is to train computer programs with human-like intellect. For this, AI uses computers to learn human behaviors, such as learning, judgment, and decision-making by simulating human intelligent behavior with computers. The term artificial intelligence was first proposed in 1956 at a conference at Dartmouth University; however, the major AI-related research started since the end of the twentieth century. AI has provided enormous economic benefits to humanity and has helped all parts of life, while also considerably promoted social growth and ushered in a new era of social development [16, 17]. Both the volume and the multidimensionality of data have increased dramatically as a result of the advent of numerous high-throughput technologies. Big data is both a requirement and a key component for AI to improve its recognition rate and accuracy [16].

Machine learning (ML), a branch of AI, is the use of an algorithm that improves its performance by learning from data. Machine learning, according to Arthur Samuel, is described as a computer's ability to analyze without being explicitly programmed [16, 18]. Supervised learning, unsupervised learning, semisupervised learning, and reinforcement learning are the four types of machine learning algorithms [16]. In supervised learning, the test data are trained with a labeled dataset to predict the type or value of new data, whereas unsupervised learning uses unlabeled data based on the input pattern. Support vector machine (SVM), linear discrimination, and decision tree are some of the types of supervised learning algorithms, whereas k-clustering and principal component analysis are the examples of unsupervised learning algorithms. Semisupervised learning combines the benefits of both supervised and unsupervised learning. It can be useful if there exist unlabeled data and collecting the labeled data is a time-consuming procedure. Reinforcement learning seeks to solve a problem through a hit-and-trial strategy, including feedback and decisions, with the ultimate goal of increasing total reward [16, 18, 19]. Deep learning (DL), a subset of machine learning, is one of the most cutting-edge areas of research and development in practically every scientific and technical discipline. Many problems that normal ML algorithms could not solve, such as image recognition and speech recognition, can be solved with the help of DL methods. DL methods also have immense role in the drug discovery pipelines, including drug activity prediction, target identification, and lead molecule discovery. The foundations of DL are frequently implicated in neural network systems, where they are employed to develop systems capable of complicated data recognition, interpretation, and production [20].

3. AI and ML in protein structure modeling

Drug design is based on the idea of creating compounds with a regulated interaction profile against a variety of target and off-target proteins in an organism. To understand the mode of action of a candidate drug, three-dimensional (3D) details are of paramount importance. Despite the availability of a variety of experimental methods to decipher the 3D structure of proteins, such as X-ray crystallography, nuclear magnetic resonance (NMR), and cryo-electron microscopy, the sequence–structure gap, in which protein sequences vastly outnumber the number of corresponding 3D structures, frequently causes problems. In such cases, protein structure prediction methods come as a remedy [21, 22].

Over the past 30 years, AI and ML methods have been used to predict protein structure. AI programs have helped to assess and identify most accurate models. To compare the predicted models to known crystal structures, these programs are trained utilizing numerous numerically represented atomic parameters from the models, such as bond lengths, inter-residue interactions, physiochemical properties, and so on. The Critical Assessment of Protein Structure Prediction (CASP) contests have been held biannually since 1994 for the blind evaluation of cutting-edge methods for predicting three-dimensional (3D) protein structures from protein sequences [23, 24]. For the cases where a template is not available for modeling, two approaches are considered: fragment-based assembly and *ab initio* folding. Fragment-based assembly is advantageous than *ab initio* folding due to its higher accuracy and higher capability [25].

With near-experimental precision, Alphabet's DeepMind won the 13th edition of CASP in 2018 with its latest artificial intelligence (AI) system, AlphaFold [25]. The 3D structure prediction by assembling the most probable fragments by AlphaFold is done by using co-evolution analysis of a multiple sequence alignment and using deep neural networks (DNNs) to discover coevolutionary patterns in protein sequences as contact distributions and transform them into protein-specific statistical energy potentials [23]. DeepFragLib, a fragment library constructed utilizing deep contextual learning techniques to give high-quality, native-like fragments for every segment

S. No.	Tools	Description	Web-link
1	AlphaFold [26]	Protein structure prediction using AI	https://github.com/deepmind/alphafold
2	DeepFragLib [27]	Fragment library construction software by DNN	https://github.com/ElwynWang/DeepFragLib
3	ProQ3/ProQ3D [28]	Protein quality assessment using deep learning	https://proq3.bioinfo.se/
4	QACon [29]	Protein model quality assessment using ML techniques	https://swmath.org/software/34249
5	DeepQA [30]	Protein model quality assessment using deep belief networks	https://swmath.org/software/15927
6	DEFMap [31]	DL-based method for extracting the dynamics associated with atomic fluctuations concealed in cryo-EM density maps	https://github.com/clinfo/DEFMap

Table 1.
Few examples of applications of AI–ML methods in protein structure methods.

of a protein for the efficient assembly of near-native conformations, is another example of AI breakthrough in the field of structure prediction. **Table 1** represent applications of some AI-ML approaches for protein structure prediction/quality assessment.

4. ML and AI in physiochemical property calculation

In the biopharmaceutical sectors, the effective and precise forecasting of molecular characteristics of drug compounds is indeed a fundamental component of rationalized compound synthesis. Current techniques span from basic atom summation through bond energy additions, paired interatomic configurations, and more sophisticated machine learning systems capable of representing aggregate reactions among several particles or bonds. In addition, simple correlation force fields show predictive performance comparable to reference energy sources determined utilizing density functional theory with hybrid exchange-correlation functional for steady-state geometric models; even so, properly accounting for the collaborative many-body connections is required for advancing the "magic formula" of compound accuracy of 1 kcal/mol for both the steady-state and out-of-equilibrium topologies [32]. In the years 2010–2012, the initial machine learning (ML) methods for molecular modeling relied on tiny datasets with quantum mechanical (QM) features for 102–103 molecule systems. It is believed that the chemical compound space has 1060–10,100 molecular systems. Chemical spaces have grown in size and complexity during the previous decade. Data are being generated at an astonishing rate owing to large-scale QM and MD methodologies, as well as developments in high-throughput studies [33].

Machine learning models predict small molecule's properties based on their chemical structure. Because of their ease of interpretation and effectiveness on small datasets, linear models were initially used. However, over time, nonlinear models were developed to capture more complex relationships between structure and activity. The nonlinear approaches include support vector machines, recursive partitioning methods, and deep learning methods. With the availability of standardized large-scale data, deep-learning-based techniques for ADMET (absorption, distribution, metabolism, excretion, and toxicity) prediction are showing growing promise and utility. The ability to identify small compounds with increased efficacy, safety, and dosage is considerably aided by understanding ADMET characteristics. In terms of consistency and predictive performance, the graph convolutional DNN (GCNN) technique is proposed to be superior to existing approaches such as random forest (RF), Cubist, and support vector machine (SVM) for calculating ADMET characteristics [34]. The AI-based ADMET predictors utilize cellular permeability data from a diverse class of molecules generated by different cell lines. To predict acid dissociation constant of compounds, artificial neural network (ANN)-based models, graph kernels, and kernel-ridge-based models have been used. To predict the solubility of the compounds, undirected graph recursive neural networks and GCNN have been used. GCNN methods are also used to predict cytotoxicity, which is one of the important properties used in drug discovery to avoid toxic effects [35]. The latest ANN studies support immunoinformatics and chemoinformatics analysis for novel vaccine and drug discovery [11]. Examples of the AI-based tools for molecular property calculation are DeepTox (www.bioinf.jku.at/research/DeepTox), Chemputer (https://zenodo.org/record/1481731), and ORGANIC (https://github.com/aspuru-guzik-group/ORGANIC) [35].

5. ML and AI in bioactivity prediction

In order to prioritize compounds for synthesis and/or biological evaluation, quantitative structure-activity relationship (QSAR) modeling has been used [36]. The goal of QSAR models is to find a mathematical relationship between the physicochemical qualities of substances, which are represented by molecular descriptors, and their biological activity. These models are important in drug optimization because they provide a preliminary *in silico* assessment of key qualities such as activity, selectivity, and toxicity of candidate compounds. In QSAR modeling, AI/ML techniques (such as RF, SVM, Naïve Bayesian, and ANN) have been widely used. Among these techniques, the RF algorithm has been regarded as a gold standard in QSAR studies [23]. In the case of bioactivity prediction, DL approaches have shown improved performance compared with ML [35]. Few examples of AI-based tools to determine bioactivity are WDL-RF (integration of DL and RF) (https://zhanglab.ccmb.med.umich.edu/WDL-RF/), pairwiseMKL (multiple-kernel-learning-based method) (https://github.com/aalto-ics-kepaco), and DeepMalaria [37] (DL based).

6. ML and AI in drug–target interactions

To fully comprehend a drug's efficacy and usefulness, it is important to determine how it interacts with a receptor or target. Drug-protein interactions have recently been a hot topic in drug repurposing research [38]. ML algorithms have become the advanced approach for estimation of drug–target interactions due to the huge amount of obtainable drugs and target information in huge datasets, advancing as well as innovative computer networking, and inherent characteristics of different types of deep learning. A vast number of proteins have indeed been sequenced, and numerous molecules have now been synthesized since the advent of sequencing technology, high-throughput technologies, and computer-aided drug design methods. Actual information has been organized, and multiple databases have been developed based

S. No.	Tools	Description	Web-link
1	Ligdream [41]	For *de novo* drug design through generative shape-based neural network decoding	https://playmolecule.com/LigDream/
2	WADDAICA [40]	Uses both deep learning model and classical algorithms for drug design	https://heisenberg.ucam.edu:5000/
3	MolAICal [42]	Uses both deep learning model and classical algorithms for drug design	https://molaical.github.io/
4	OpenChem [39]	A deep learning toolkit for computational chemistry	https://github.com/Mariewelt/OpenChem
5	DeepAffinity [43]	A combination of RNN and CNN methods for ligand–protein affinity	https://github.com/Shen-Lab/DeepAffinity
6	DeepFrag [44]	Uses deep CNN for fragment-based lead optimization	https://durrantlab.pitt.edu/deepfragmodel/

Table 2.
Few examples of applications of AI–ML methods in drug–protein interactions.

on existing related efforts and acquired expertise. The majority of data in these sources is open to the public and free to download, thus providing a strong data basis for using deep learning to solve drug-target contact predictions issues. PubChem presently comprises 109 million chemicals and is the world's biggest database with open access to chemical characterization. PubChem has grown in importance as a source of chemical knowledge for researchers, learners, and the general public. Artificial intelligence can be used to train deep learning models for drug discovery using known drug data [39]. Several ML techniques have been used to predict drug–target interactions including SVM, DL, DNN, convolutional neural network (CNN), etc. The *de novo* drug design approach has been frequently employed to create therapeutic compounds in recent years. The old approach of *de novo* drug design is being phased out in favor of emerging DL methodologies, which have the advantages of less complicated synthesis routes and easier prediction of novel molecule bioactivity [35]. However, classical algorithms cannot be completely ignored, as studies point out that the classical algorithms show higher and more stable performance than the machine-learning-based methods at different similarity levels of training sets. Hence, many tools have been developed combining both classical and deep learning models [40]. Few of the tools and servers available for finding drug-protein interactions using AI and ML methods are mentioned in **Table 2**.

7. Conclusion

Although AI is frequently portrayed as a magic wand that can provide flawless output regardless of the quality of the input, it is not the solution to every problem. The ultimate goal of using AI and machine learning approaches to drug development challenges is to bring the best drugs to market. Throughout the drug discovery process, the combined effort of different AI methods allows for a better understanding and design of novel inputs [45]. The AI-based applications are getting more intelligent, cost-effective, and time-efficient while increasing efficacy, because of more precise algorithms, more powerful supercomputers, and significant private and public investment in the sector [20]. To properly leverage AI in drug development, one must increase the quality of decisions we make regarding compounds that are progressed to clinical trials. However, in many circumstances, the data available to make those decisions are not totally sufficient for this purpose [46]. Since the entire success of AI depends on the availability of a substantial amount of data, we need to conduct trials more efficiently, which can be supported by computational methods [35, 46]. Major challenges faced by AI methods include data accuracy and availability, reproducibility, model appropriateness, etc. Despite the challenges, AI is projected to advance the field of personalized/precision medicine to the point where it becomes regular practice even in the treatment of minor illnesses in the future [47]. By 2028, AI is expected to save the pharmaceutical industry more than US$70 billion in drug discovery costs [48]. With more clinical data and improved AI calculations, AI is projected to improve many elements of drug discovery and development and will eventually become the standard computer-assisted technique for drug discovery.

Acknowledgements

ANJ would like to acknowledge Department of Science and Technology (DST-SERB File no. CRG/2020/001829), Government of India, for providing computational facilities.

Author details

Subhomoi Borkotoky[1*], Amit Joshi[1,2], Vikas Kaushik[2] and Anupam Nath Jha[3*]

1 Department of Biotechnology, Invertis University, Bareilly, UP, India

2 School of Bio-Engineering and Bio-Sciences, Lovely Professional University, Phagwara, Punjab, India

3 Department of Molecular Biology and Biotechnology, Tezpur University, Tezpur, Assam, India

*Address all correspondence to: drsubhomoi.b@invertis.org and anjha@tezu.ernet.in

References

[1] Das A et al. *Plasmodium falciparum*: Experimental and theoretical approaches in last 20 years. In: Current Topics and Emerging Issues in Malaria Elimination. London, UK: IntechOpen; 2021

[2] Borah PK et al. In silico approaches and proportional odds model towards identifying selective ADAM17 inhibitors from anti-inflammatory natural molecules. Journal of Molecular Graphics & Modelling. 2016;**70**:129-139

[3] Maia EHB et al. Structure-based virtual screening: From classical to artificial intelligence. Frontiers in Chemistry. 2020;**8**:343

[4] Baig MH et al. Computer aided drug design and its application to the development of potential drugs for neurodegenerative disorders. Current Neuropharmacology. 2018;**16**(6):740-748

[5] Jakhmola S et al. In silico analysis of antiviral phytochemicals efficacy against Epstein–Barr virus glycoprotein H. Journal of Biomolecular Structure and Dynamics. 2021:1-14

[6] Hazarika Z, Jha AN. Computational analysis of the silver nanoparticle–human serum albumin complex. ACS Omega. 2020;**5**(1):170-178

[7] Mirza SB et al. Virtual screening of eighteen million compounds against dengue virus: Combined molecular docking and molecular dynamics simulations study. Journal of Molecular Graphics & Modelling. 2016;**66**:99-107

[8] Borkotoky S et al. Identification of high affinity and low molecular alternatives of boceprevir against SARS-CoV-2 main protease: A virtual screening approach. Chemical Physics Letters. 2021;**770**:138446

[9] Hazarika Z, Rajkhowa S, Jha AN. Role of Force Fields in Protein Function Prediction. Croatia: IntechOpen; 2020

[10] Rajkhowa S, Hazarika Z, Jha AN. Systems biology and bioinformatics approaches in leishmaniasis. In: Applications of Nanobiotechnology for Neglected Tropical Diseases. Academic Press: United States; 2021. pp. 509-548

[11] Borah SM, Jha AN. Identification and analysis of structurally critical fragments in HopS2. BMC Bioinformatics. 2019;**19**(Suppl. 13):552

[12] Bora N, Jha AN. An integrative approach using systems biology, mutational analysis with molecular dynamics simulation to challenge the functionality of a target protein. Chemical Biology & Drug Design. 2019;**93**(6):1050-1060

[13] Das S et al. Exploring the interaction of bioactive kaempferol with serum albumin, lysozyme and hemoglobin: A biophysical investigation using multi-spectroscopic, docking and molecular dynamics simulation studies. Journal of Photochemistry and Photobiology B: Biology. 2020;**205**(111825)

[14] Gentile F et al. Artificial intelligence-enabled virtual screening of ultra-large chemical libraries with deep docking. Nature Protocols. 2022;672-697

[15] Hazarika Z, Jha AN. A comparative evaluation of docking programs using influenza endonuclease as target protein. In: 2020 International Conference on Computational Performance Evaluation (ComPE). 2020

[16] Zhang C, Lu Y. Study on artificial intelligence: The state of the art and

future prospects. Journal of Industrial Information Integration. 2021;**23**:100224

[17] Das S et al. Applications of artificial intelligence in machine learning: Review and prospect. International Journal of Computer Applications. 2015;**115**(9):31-41

[18] Kaur G, Goyal S, Kaur H. Brief Review of Various Machine Learning Algorithms. In: Proceedings of the International Conference on Innovative Computing & Communication (ICICC). 2021;1-8

[19] Mahesh B. Machine learning algorithms—A review. International Journal of Science and Research. 2020;**9**:381-386

[20] Patel L et al. Machine learning methods in drug discovery. Molecules. 2020;**25**(22):1-17

[21] Schmidt T, Bergner A, Schwede T. Modelling three-dimensional protein structures for applications in drug design. Drug Discovery Today. 2014;**19**:890-897

[22] Rajkhowa S et al. Design of Plasmodium falciparum PI(4)KIIIβ Inhibitor using Molecular Dynamics and Molecular Docking Methods. ChemistrySelect. 2017;**2**:1783-1792

[23] Vatansever S et al. Artificial intelligence and machine learning-aided drug discovery in central nervous system diseases: State-of-the-arts and future directions. Medicinal Research Reviews. 2021;**41**(3):1427-1473

[24] Staples M et al. Artificial intelligence for bioinformatics: Applications in protein folding prediction. In: 2019 IEEE Technology & Engineering Management Conference (TEMSCON); IEEE. 2019

[25] Wei G-W. Protein structure prediction beyond AlphaFold. Nature Machine Intelligence. 2019;**1**(8):336-337

[26] Jumper J et al. Highly accurate protein structure prediction with AlphaFold. Nature. 2021;**596**(7873): 583-589

[27] Wang T et al. Improved fragment sampling for ab initio protein structure prediction using deep neural networks. Nature Machine Intelligence. 2019;**1**(8):347-355

[28] Uziela K et al. ProQ3D: Improved model quality assessments using deep learning. Bioinformatics. 2017;**33**(10):1578-1580

[29] Cao R et al. QAcon: Single model quality assessment using protein structural and contact information with machine learning techniques. Bioinformatics. 2016;**33**(4):586-588

[30] Cao R et al. DeepQA: Improving the estimation of single protein model quality with deep belief networks. BMC Bioinformatics. 2016;**17**(1):495

[31] Matsumoto S et al. Extraction of protein dynamics information from cryo-EM maps using deep learning. Nature Machine Intelligence. 2021;**3**(2):153-160

[32] Hansen K et al. Machine learning predictions of molecular properties: Accurate many-body potentials and nonlocality in chemical space. The Journal of Physical Chemistry Letters. 2015;**6**(12):2326-2331

[33] Karthikeyan A, Priyakumar UD. Artificial intelligence: Machine learning for chemical sciences. Journal of Chemical Sciences (Bangalore). 2022;**134**(1):2

[34] Caceres EL, Tudor M, Cheng AC. Deep learning approaches in predicting

ADMET properties. Future Medicinal Chemistry. 2020;**12**(22):1995-1999

[35] Paul D et al. Artificial intelligence in drug discovery and development. Drug Discovery Today. 2021;**26**(1):80-93

[36] Neves BJ et al. QSAR-based virtual screening: Advances and applications in drug discovery. Frontiers in Pharmacology. 2018;**9**:1-7

[37] Keshavarzi Arshadi A et al. DeepMalaria: Artificial intelligence driven discovery of potent antiplasmodials. Frontiers in Pharmacology. 2020;**10**:1-13

[38] Wang W et al. DLS: A link prediction method based on network local structure for predicting drug–protein interactions. Frontiers in Bioengineering and Biotechnology. 2020;**8**:330

[39] Korshunova M et al. OpenChem: A deep learning toolkit for computational chemistry and drug design. Journal of Chemical Information and Modeling. 2021;**61**(1):7-13

[40] Bai Q et al. WADDAICA: A webserver for aiding protein drug design by artificial intelligence and classical algorithm. Computational and Structural Biotechnology Journal. 2021;**19**:3573-3579

[41] Skalic M et al. Shape-based generative modeling for de novo drug design. Journal of Chemical Information and Modeling. 2019;**59**(3):1205-1214

[42] Bai Q et al. MolAICal: A soft tool for 3D drug design of protein targets by artificial intelligence and classical algorithm. Briefings in Bioinformatics. 2020;**22**(3)

[43] Karimi M et al. DeepAffinity: Iinterpretable deep learning of compound–protein affinity through unified recurrent and convolutional neural networks. Bioinformatics. 2019;**35**(18):3329-3338

[44] Green H, Koes DR, Durrant JD. DeepFrag: A deep convolutional neural network for fragment-based lead optimization. Chemical Science. 2021;**12**(23):8036-8047

[45] Sellwood MA et al. Artificial intelligence in drug discovery. Future Medicinal Chemistry. 2018;**10**(17):2025-2028

[46] Bender A, Cortes-Ciriano I. Artificial intelligence in drug discovery: What is realistic, what are illusions? Part 2: A discussion of chemical and biological data. Drug Discovery Today. 2021;**26**(4):1040-1052

[47] Arabi AA. Artificial intelligence in drug design: Algorithms, applications, challenges and ethics. Future Drug Discovery. 2021;**3**(2):FDD59

[48] Piekarz D. AI in Drug Development: A Glimpse Into the Future of Drug Discovery. 2021. Available from: https://www.dataart.com/blog/ai-in-drug-development-a-glimpse-into-the-future-of-drug-discovery